*Tammy,
Thank You
much for the
Best peace
happiness ♡ Dinee*

Eating Light, Done Right

Eating Light, Done Right

Simply Sinless Recipes from the Single Mom Next Door

TANIA N. BOUGHTON

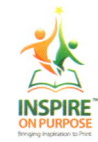

INSPIRE
ON PURPOSE
Bringing Inspiration to Print

Published by Inspire On Purpose™
909 Lake Carolyn Parkway, Suite 300
Irving, Texas 75039
Toll Free 888-403-2727
www.inspireonpurpose.com
The Platform Publisher™

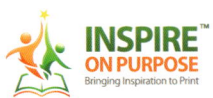

Printed in the United States of America

Library of Congress Control Number: 2011944805

ISBN 10: 0982562233
ISBN 13: 978-0-9825622-3-9

Table of Contents

A Note from the Author:

There are many things in this world I have sought to become, however a "victim" was never one of them. In writing this book, I reveal many things that have occurred throughout the course of my life; ups, downs and the turmoil of agonizing decisions and daily struggles. Very, very few people know about much of this drama including my own family. There are several people in my life that I don't even want to read this book, because pieces of the story are emotionally charged, embarrassing and difficult to discuss. The majority of my friends don't even know I struggled with weight problems, emotional eating or the demons of bad relationships. To these people, I have painted a picture of strength and Camelot, because having witnessed poverty, true suffering and the deaths of friends, I myself have never yearned for sympathy.

"The world breaks everyone, and afterward, some are strong in the broken places..." Ernest Hemingway

I've shared my story in the hopes that everyone who reads it realizes that they too can be strong in the broken places.

~ *Tania*

A part of the proceeds from the sale of *Eating Light, Done Right* will be donated to the Cystic Fibrosis Foundation, a cause that is near and dear to my heart. Please visit my website for more information about how to support this charity. **www.EatingLightDoneRight.com**

Acknowledgements

First, I have so many people to thank that I can't possibly list them all, but to those of you who know who you are...Thank you!

Funny thing about those two simple words. They can never be said enough, and they have the most profound impact on people.

In addition, I want to say thank you...

To my sons, Tristan and Tanner, my inspiration for the book, and my motivation in life. You are my most precious treasures.

To my family, especially my parents, who after more than thirty years are still hopelessly in love. My father instilled in me a work ethic like no other while my mother and sisters held up the pom-poms, even when I wasn't in the mood for cheering.

To Mike, for being my rock and for showing me the meaning of love, respect and trust...and for loving me in the unlovable moments as well as the loveable ones.

To Tammy, my truest and dearest friend, thank you for believing in me, accepting my flaws and for never leaving me.

To Amanda, whom I think about every day as I look at her picture in my kitchen. It's in her memory that I continue to raise money and awareness for cystic fibrosis.

To Natalie, for daring me to dream, for walking the talk and for being my biggest fan.

To Randy, for hearing a little story from the girl next door and pushing me off the ledge to actually DO this! Thank you for believing in me.

To my sweet friend Eunice at Marmalade Days photography, thank you so much for capturing my boys in the kitchen so perfectly. I will cherish these pictures and memories forever.

To Marc, for being a friend and for lending your expert advice in the gym so we don't hurt ourselves messing with things we can't pronounce.

To the gals at Inspire, Michelle and Terri, thank you for drinking the Kool-Aid, for having "my back," and for turning the words of this book into a true piece of art.

To my team at J. Hilburn, were it not for them and this career, I would not have time to pursue these dreams of mine. Who knew that a career in men's custom fashion would be the gateway to changing my life?

Thank you also to all the people over the years who've come to me for help and asked me how I lost the weight and kept it off. What tremendous motivation to know that I can help so many people.

Finally, thank you to God...the Man upstairs...It is my faith that guides me and continues to shine the light.

Every day, I read two quotes I keep on my marker board in front of me. The first, "I can do all things in Him who strengthens me," reminds me daily to have faith and to walk "heart first" and with grace on the narrow path, trying to be mindful of everyone I meet along the way.

I'll leave you to work my final quote into your own life as you see fit, because it truly applies to everyone: "It is never too late to become what you might have been."

Thank you, thank you, thank you, and here's to becoming what we all might be.

Hugs,

~ *Tania*

Section 1:

Get the Big Picture

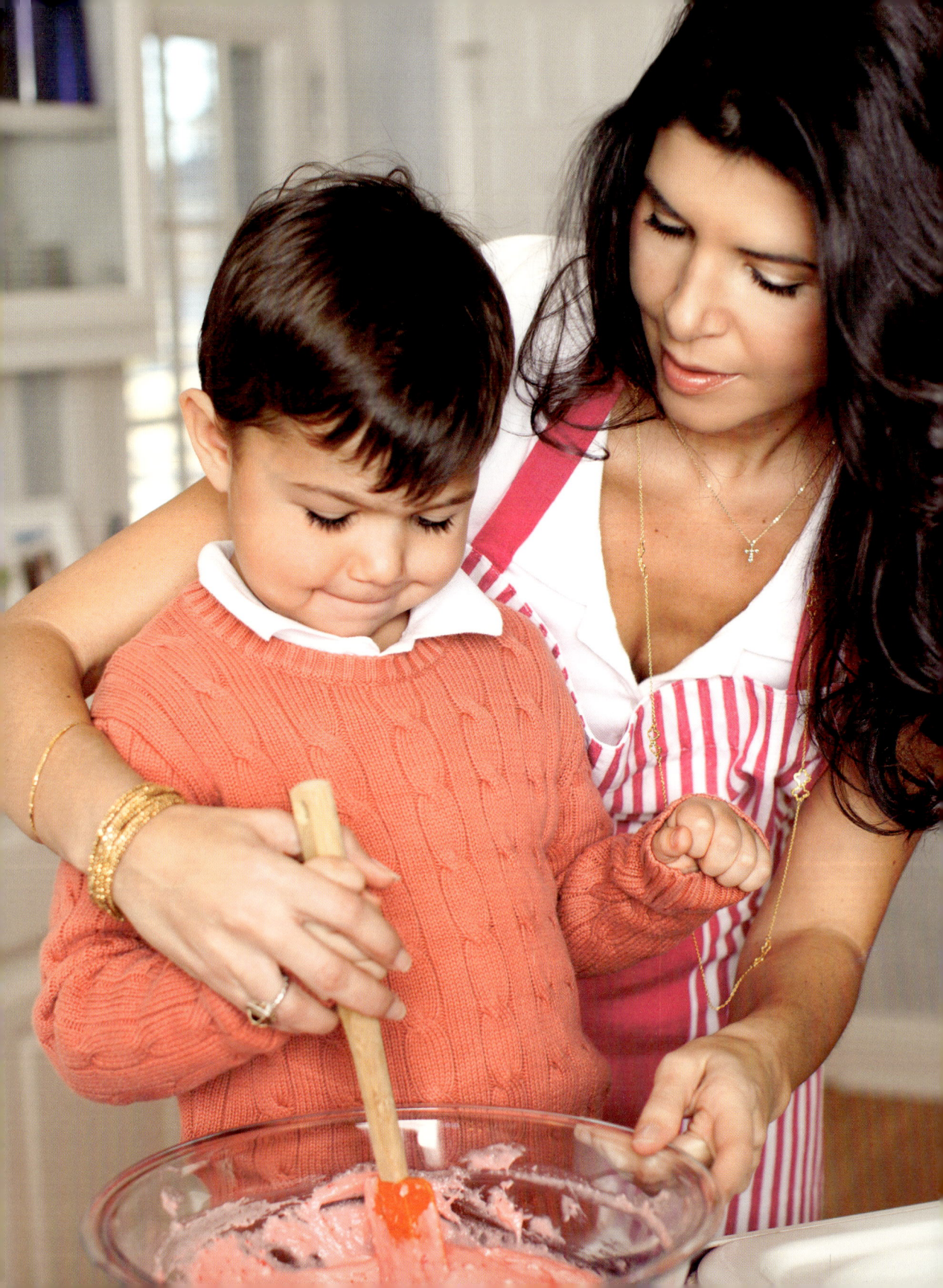

Chapter 1:
Another Big Girl Moment

In the beginning, I was fat. There are more politically correct ways to describe myself as a big girl, but the voice in my head kept repeating the phrase, "You are fat, you are fat, you are fat."

I could begin my story anywhere, but I'll start at the exact point when I realized my life had once again spun out of control – when I sought solace in a jar of Nutella while standing on a scale two weeks after the birth of my second son.

You know Nutella, right? That creamy hazelnut and chocolate mixture sent as manna from Heaven? I loved opening that jar with the unsuspicious white label, the immediate whiff of chocolaty, nutty goodness filling my nostrils, the scent alone making my mouth water.

I'd just slathered it all over one of those obnoxious 750-calorie croissants from Costco. You know, the ones that come in an eight-pack? I was still holding the jar of Nutella when I walked over to the scale and lumbered on.

To my horror, I weighed in at 203 pounds. Truly, I couldn't believe my eyes. I'd stopped weighing myself two weeks prior to giving birth, having convinced myself the fat would melt as soon as I began nursing, and I'd had no idea I'd gained so much.

Realizing I was fifty-plus pounds heavier than my normal weight two weeks after giving birth was demoralizing and humiliating, and surely it didn't bode well for the quality of my life going forward, or that of my children. Even as I reached into the jar of Nutella one last time, I thought, "This can't go on."

I was faced with the daunting task of stripping off this weight. I knew I'd eaten myself into oblivion. I knew the health risks of obesity. I knew my family carried diabetic tendencies. I knew I'd never be able to keep up with my children at this weight. Above all, I knew if I didn't do something NOW, I never would.

The even uglier truth I needed to confront was why I'd gained all this weight in the first place. That harsh reality was weighing on my heart like a year's worth of buttered croissants dipped in anything chocolate. I had become an emotional eater...again. The question was,

How did I get here?

As a child, I wasn't overweight by any stretch. In fact, I was an athlete. As a swimmer, I worked out so much that I could eat anything I wanted and still maintain my muscular frame. But as I grew up and out of swimming, I slowly realized I was following in the footsteps of my family and countless others using food as a coping mechanism to deal with the stresses of life.

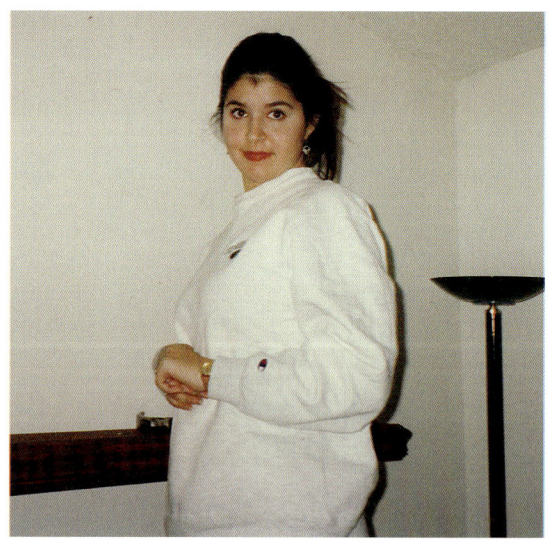

Age 21. In unhappier times at 210 lbs. (Size 16)

As a young adult on my own for the first time, I found my eating decisions quickly beginning to slide as I endured the emotional roller coaster of a difficult relationship. This was infuriating, because I had the tools in my toolbox to stay fit and healthy.

I'd joined the service at age seventeen, and the Army had taught me many things, including how to exercise to maximum efficiency. The fact was, I was perfectly capable of cooking healthy meals and exercising to stay fit and healthy, yet I lacked two crucial elements that absolutely sank my ship: willpower and self-control.

I only stopped eating junk when my weight ballooned (literally) to 205 pounds and I realized what I was doing to myself. I began exercising with a girlfriend and cooking healthfully, and I regained my self-control. To my delight, I lost forty pounds in three months.

Shortly thereafter, I ended my problematic relationship and moved back to Texas, where I began my collegiate career on the GI Bill and managed the Weight Management program for my National Guard unit. Ironically, I found myself counseling numerous troops on the effects of poor eating decisions and the strain on every aspect of their lives, including their careers, their relationships and their health. As I knew all too well, there's not one single area of life that isn't negatively impacted by continuing to remain overweight.

Meanwhile, I began another bad relationship. This individual was so concerned about the possibility that I might regain my former weight that he asked me daily if I'd worked out, questioned what I ate, and at one point told me I had the "potential" to become a "hot chick turned fatty."

Shortly thereafter, he informed me that he and his friends had decided I could be a victim of B.A.N.T.'S disease (Big A$$ No T's) if I wasn't careful and didn't keep my rear in check. What a peach, eh?

Again, I began letting the sorrow of a bad relationship seep in. Only this time, I refused to gain weight out of fear of having another failed relationship. So instead, I LOST weight...rapidly. I worked out maniacally and counted every calorie I consumed to the point that I actually attempted to burn more calories via exercise than I'd consumed in the day.

I ate as "low fat" as possible and the results were not pretty: my hair became brittle, my hipbones and collarbone jutted out from my frame, and finally my periods stopped. This was my wake-up call. I was twenty-five years old, stood 5'11," and weighed 122 pounds when my body stopped functioning as a female.

I was at ground zero, with another relationship down the toilet, struggling with another period in time that I coped with poorly and emotionally through food – this time, by all but rejecting it. I remember thinking to myself, "At some point this will stop...right?"

Fast-forward two years to my senior year in college. I was casually dating someone and was about to begin exams. I wasn't feeling well in the mornings and a glance at the calendar sent a shotgun blast through my life.

I was pregnant...I couldn't be pregnant...I had my packet in for the Army's Officer Candidate School in Austin...I was close to graduating...the "relationship" was entirely too new...we weren't even exclusive. Yet there I was, due to have a son in December of 2003 and forced to withdraw from school as the pregnancy was very difficult and I couldn't keep my head out of the commode.

I decided that marriage was not an option and would only make a difficult situation worse; however we did decide to attempt a relationship and stayed together for several years. I knew that the arrival of this little boy would change everything and he would be the center of my universe. I can't even have hindsight and say I shouldn't have attempted to make the relationship work, because then I wouldn't have my second son. For me, my boys were the silver linings in a sky full of storm clouds.

Three years later, now living in a different state, I continued to try to make the best of our circumstances, but they were tumultuous at best. The boys' father and I had different ideas of what family life looked like, and so he worked on chasing his big dreams, waking early and retiring late, barely home, and when home, angry.

Every day became an exercise in walking on eggshells. Although we had a few ups, they were far outweighed by the downs, and I learned to be a "single" mom early in our relationship. I worked, supported our family and ran the household, but this only made things more difficult in the long run and in fact built resentment and more anger in him.

Again I turned to food for comfort. I loved eating out at the local Chinese restaurant and grabbing fatty, easy foods from the hot food bar at our local market. Slowly the weight began to creep back on, meal by meal, inch by inch. I was in a holding pattern, juggling a successful real estate career and motherhood while futilely attempting to keep a doomed relationship together.

I decided that a second baby would repair things, but almost immediately upon conceiving my second precious son, I realized my relationship with his father was circling the drain.

Again I turned to food, this time with a vengeance, pregnancy being my excuse to consume anything and everything in my path. I was a woman on a mission...to drown myself in anything soft, sugary and sweet. I found solace in the baked goods aisle and actually became excited about the morning breakfast drive-thru!

So here we are, full circle, back to the scale. I stood there gawking, still holding that jar of Nutella. The croissant, sad to say, I'd already devoured. Could I really be fifty-three pounds over my normal weight two weeks after delivering this amazing baby? Why in fact did I keep doing this to myself?

I was in agony and it took me some hard thinking to finally figure out that,

It's all about self-love

Truth be told, I didn't love myself, and I didn't think I was worthy of happiness in a relationship. If I were fat, I had an excuse for why no one wanted me, one that didn't have anything to do with what all those men I'd dated had conditioned me to believe.

Over the years, the men I dated in the past had essentially told me I was stupid, stubborn, emotional, headstrong, crazy, judgmental and too independent, with nothing going for me but a pretty face that would fail as I aged.

I listened to these words for years and put up with taunting from old boyfriends and their friends until finally, on this particular day, I cracked. I wasn't crazy, but finding out that a boyfriend was unfaithful, treated me like I was disposable, preferred to spend his time in bars and at certain glittery clubs than at home with me was enough to make anyone just a little batty. We've all dated this guy, it was time to stop being embarrassed and realize he was wrong in both his opinions and treatment of me.

What did I tell myself? That I'm not crazy, and I'm certainly not stupid – I'm just educated in areas that interest me. I admit, I really don't know much about foreign policy, but if you need to treat a sucking chest wound, then call me.

Yes, I'm independent and I love my routine. I like alone time in the mornings to drink my tea, check emails and watch Charles Osgood on Sunday mornings because I adore him and his show. I need alone time for exercise, Yoga and occasionally I like to take a bath… there's nothing wrong with that.

Stubborn? Sometimes, but typically only over black and white issues.

Emotional? You betcha. I also give money to every homeless person I see, raise money for local charities, host fundraisers, and am the first person my friends call when in crisis. Being "emotional" isn't a bad thing, and it's enabled me to be a more empathetic person.

Headstrong? Sometimes, but I'd rather have an opinion than regret not speaking up.

The list continued as I talked myself out of this hole I'd been buried in for years. I was none of these unflattering things I'd been told I was to any significant degree. On the contrary, I was a good, kind-hearted, loving person. I was worthy of a happy, fulfilling relationship because I was beginning to love myself, and one day, someone would love all the bad along with all the good about me. Emotional eater NO MORE. Loving myself was the start of the new and improved version of Tania.

On that very day, I made the decision to stop the cycle, get the weight off quickly, keep it off, maintain records of all my recipes and help others do the same. Today, without any doubt whatsoever, I know that…

If I can do it, so can you

It is my sincerest hope that by chronicling my musings, discoveries and opinions about food, cooking and exercise that I can take the intimidation out of cooking healthfully. I truly AM the single mother who lives next door, balancing motherhood to two little boys, one of whom has Asperger's, with my career, charity work, sports schedules, PTA, exercise and life in general, all while cooking healthy meals day in and day out…Yes, I am one busy woman, and if I can do it, you can too.

Bottom line, I'm not a certified expert in anything. I'm not a professional chef, trainer, nutritionist, writer, or counselor. I've written this book from a frank, sometimes funny, always honest perspective. Honestly, if you're looking for Brontë or Dickinson, you won't find them here. What you will find is my personal approach to healthy eating – an approach that, going on five years now, has kept me slim, trim, happy and healthy, in spite of my checkered past.

What's more, there are enough recipes in the book to keep life interesting for a month at least!

I do have a few biases before we begin. Please know up-front that I don't believe in buying $500.00 worth of cookware to get started in the kitchen, and I don't have my own herb garden. If a recipe is too complicated, I don't make it, and I trust that you won't either. Cooking and eating healthfully shouldn't be difficult, and it's perfectly fine to fail in the kitchen. In fact, I burn myself constantly and more than once have turned out a disastrous dish...my two beloved sons can attest to that.

My point in sharing all this is that if I can make cooking and eating healthfully a lifetime commitment, anyone can. So let's get started!

Key points in this chapter:

- Ask yourself, *"How did I get here?"* Taking a good look at what brought you to this point in life can help you make changes.

- Remember, it takes willpower and self-control to lose weight.

- If I can do it, so can you.

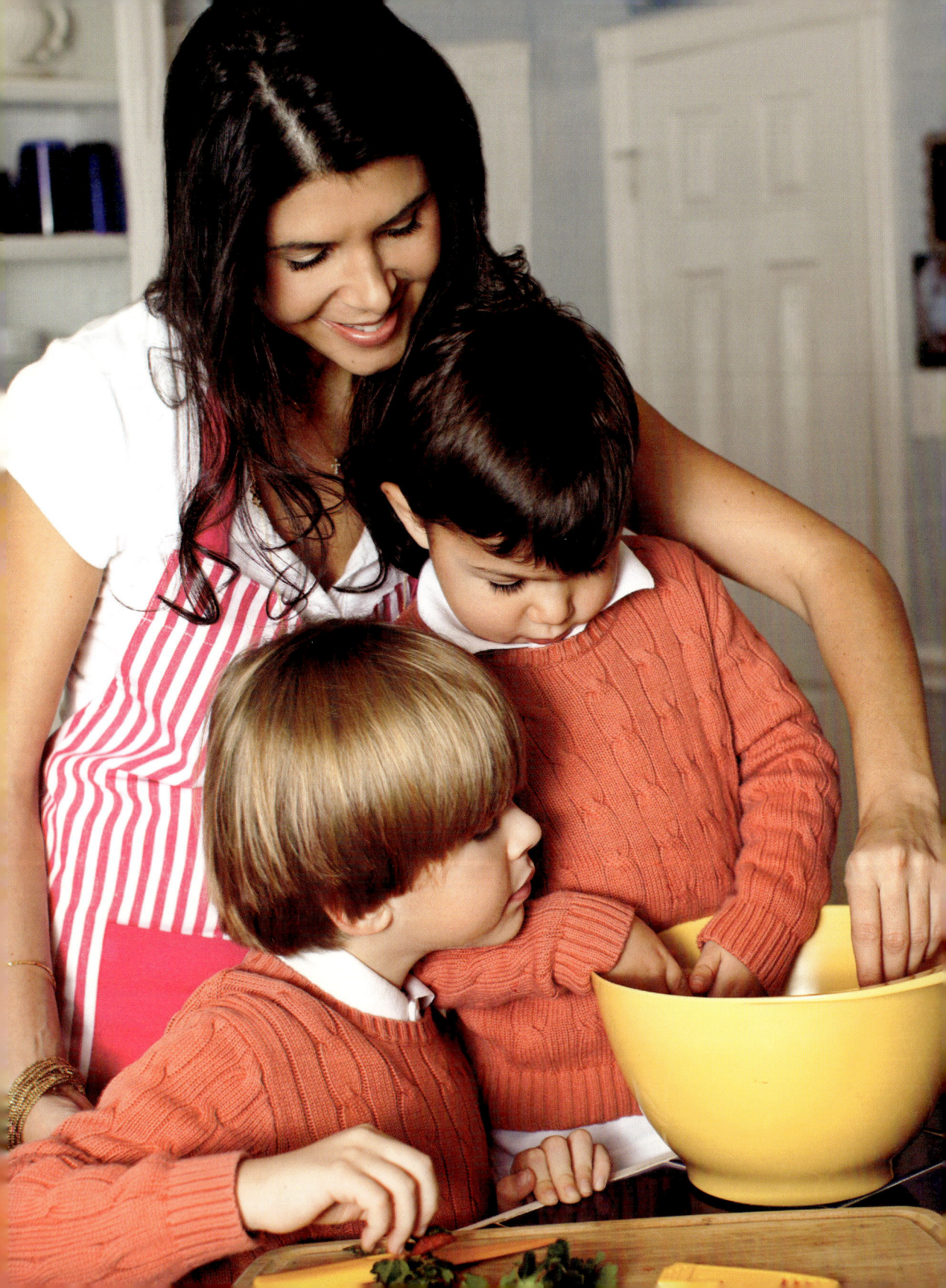

Chapter 2 :

Just Say "No" to Fad Diets

The basic premise of this chapter is simple: "If it's too complicated or scientific, doesn't taste good, or involves the eradication of an entire food group, you aren't going to stick with it."

What does this mean for you? You'll enjoy a temporary weight loss if you eat nothing but grapefruit every day, but you'll gain it all back once you've had enough of Florida's favorite citrus.

In other words, steer clear of fad diets – all of them – including the no carb, low carb, whatever you want to call it diet. In truth, the low carb diet was developed for heart surgery patients who needed to drop massive amounts of weight quickly so they could survive an operation...in many cases, a surgery necessitated by their obesity!

Cutting out all fruits, carbs and grains and replacing them with nothing but protein is also a recipe for disaster. A girlfriend of mine tried this diet and was miserable because she couldn't have tomatoes. What? No tomatoes? Who can maintain that lifestyle? Here's my bottom line:

Deprivation is not a healthy way to lose weight

Let's discuss why exactly we need carbs. I bring this up because it was a serious revelation on my part. It can be summed up in one simple word...FIBER! We need the fiber in carbs to keep our hind ends from clogging up. If we don't eat fiber, we don't flush waste and we end up a bloated, constipated mess.

I don't know about you, but a lifetime of laxatives is not an option for this gal. Stock up on complex carbs and enjoy your food.

The bottom line on the low-carb fad is this: eating only protein will result in weight loss as you do burn fat in a state of ketosis, strip your excess water weight and you drop initial pounds, but can you maintain this form of nutrition for the remainder of your life? Fast forward to three months from now as you begin eating carbs again and slowly start gaining weight. How discouraging! Furthermore, a long-term protein-only diet is not good for your heart or kidneys...skinny with kidney failure? Hmm, food for thought. Again, I'm not the expert here, however the Mayo clinic is. Look up low carb diet kidney failure and read what the experts say.

As far as I'm concerned, the veggie-only diet is just as bad as the low-carb diet. I'm not getting into a Biblical discussion on why animals are on this earth. I've heard and discussed both sides of this debate ad nauseum. I understand that a small percentage of the planet doesn't eat meat for personal reasons and that is absolutely their choice. I wholeheartedly understand because I was a vegetarian for several years. To this day, my personal meat choices are free-range chicken and turkey, moderate amounts of sushi, and kosher beef.

But back to the veggie diet...As a vegetarian, a lifestyle I embraced from for several years, I weighed 120-125 pounds and was the unhealthiest I'd ever been in my life. Replacing protein sources with lentils and cutting out dairy and meat left me bloated and dependent on Beano, a mere shell of the woman I am today. I'll be honest, I had zero energy and no muscle tone, and my mood swings were equivalent to that of a theme park roller coaster.

Maybe I didn't do it "right"...who knows? Bottom line, I was skinny, but I was too miserable to enjoy it. That's when I realized that diets that involve the complete eradication of a food group are doomed to failure.

And what about the rest of the fad diets...the all-liquid diet, the detox diet, the juice diet? Some of my friends have tried these methods to "jump start" their weight loss. I'll concede they're somewhat effective in making you feel lighter, but attempting a liquid-only diet for an extended period (longer than three to four days) is neither healthy, nor possible.

Seriously, who drinks juice for days on end and expects to keep the weight off once actual food is ingested? I know these diets are called "fat flushes," but guess what you're flushing? Everything in your body that is stored as waste from solid foods! Yes, you'll drop weight, but you'll probably spend more time on the potty than you'd like. Worst of all, as soon as you begin eating solids again, you'll begin storing again. That's just the natural process of digestion.

Use common sense and ask yourself this question: "Am I going to be able to keep this up for the rest of my life?"

If the answer is no, skip it! Instead of embracing a fad diet of any kind…

Take responsibility for your knife, fork and spoon

We all know that losing weight does not involve rocket science, just willpower. The actual formula is actually rather simple:

Eat Less + Move More = Weight Loss.

I'm not trying to be sarcastic, just very truthful. We all know how to make good choices. For example, back when my pantry was full of [insert name of any breakfast cereal seen on a Saturday morning cartoon show commercial] I KNEW I was overindulging, both at the store and at home.

I also knew I wasn't going to lose weight by continuing to eat these foods for breakfast (or for snacks, or during fits of insomnia). I had decisions to make, but it wasn't easy. Cereal companies have done a clever job of packaging their cereals to make them appear healthier than they are, with bold labels on these sugary treats screaming "whole grain!" and "1/3 LESS sugar!"

I had to steel myself not to be fooled by these marketing ploys, and you need to steel yourself to resist them as well. Let's face it: anything that is covered in sugar and surrounded by marshmallows should NOT be in your house, much less in your bowl, with milk and a spoon!

Remember, refined and processed = unhealthy! Your choices for breakfast, not to mention lunch and dinner, should revolve around whole wheat, fruit, grains, oats and lean proteins.

Of course, I realize that eating on the go can throw a wrench into anyone's best-laid plans and good intentions. It's simply time to face up to the fact that weight loss won't occur in the drive-thru. If you order the double cheeseburger wrapped in lettuce instead of a bun, you're trying to fool yourself into thinking it's a good decision because it's "low carb."

Trust me, I've been there. I have the ability to talk myself into anything. For me, it was truly shocking to realize that carbs were not the enemy. The saturated fats and oils used to make that 30% "fatburger" are what clog your arteries and put cellulite on your thighs.

Here's a tip: if you're overscheduled, overstressed and running against the clock, you're most likely to overindulge and make poor eating decisions, which lead you to become overweight.

Notice my repetitive use of the word "over"? It's an important word! Eliminating some of the "overs" in your life can be quite simple. Running short on time? Pack a meal the night before and invest in a small cooler for your car. You can be in control of what you prepare for consumption and not be a victim of the drive-thru!

On the flip side, sometimes packing your lunch every day can be annoying, and you don't always have access to your car or the cooler. If you ARE faced with restaurant or fast-food decisions, make intelligent ones. Some of my personal favorites are:

- Kung Pao Chicken at Pei Wei made "stock velvet," which means steamed with brown rice OR extra veggies

- the Chicken Burrito Bowl at Chipotle, with black beans, all the veggies possible, light cheese, NO sour cream and mild salsa for a kick

- the Asian Chicken Salad at McDonalds

- the Grilled Chicken Teriyaki Sandwich at Carl's Jr. (wrapped in lettuce to avoid the white bun)

- Chicken Soft Tacos at Taco Bell made "Ranchero" style...

Get my point? Don't get stuck in the fat rut. Do utilize your common sense and self-control. Moreover, don't let co-workers, friends or family pressure you into making poor eating decisions when you go out to eat with them. You have healthy options, and breaking the cycle begins with your self-control.

It's really quite simple: you truly are what you eat. I hope this motto resonates with you. If you're eating sugary, refined cereals for your first meal of the day, you're immediately sending your body into sugar shock and you'll LOOK like a marshmallow. Soft, gooey and puffy.

Take responsibility for what you eat, and you've taken the first step to a healthier you!

Key points in this chapter:

- Make lifetime eating decisions you can maintain.

- Remember that deprivation is not a healthy way to lose weight.

- What "overs" do you need to eliminate from your life?

- Take responsibility for your knife, fork and spoon.

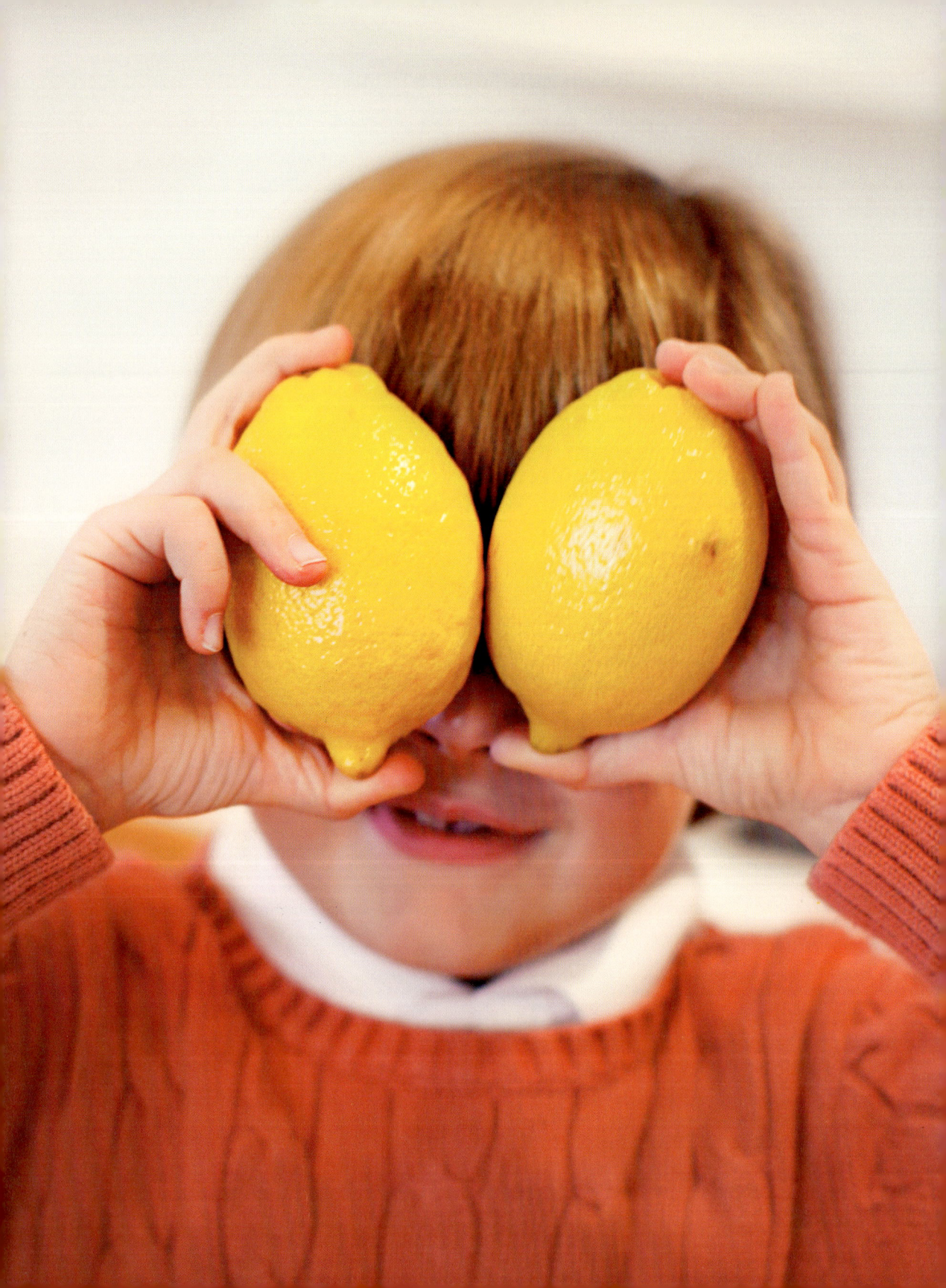

Chapter 3 :

The "Celebumom" Phenomenon

This subject might be the one I personally identify with the most and am also asked about on a near daily basis.

The number of gals who approach me when I'm working out at the gym and exclaim, "Oh my gosh! So and so got her baby weight off and was on a magazine cover [or on the runway or movie set] in just THREE months...I want HER body!" is legion. I am constantly asked the question, "How can I look like [insert name of insanely beautiful actress or actor] and get that body?"

I'd like to address a couple of obvious points about these celebrity people, the first being that they are genetically gifted, and the second...Well, it's their job to look good. It's probably not yours, and it's certainly not mine. These leading actors make millions of dollars because they are marketable and everyone wants to "be" like them.

Now look in the mirror. How tall are you? What do your muscles look like? Are they long and lean, or smaller and more compact? What is your body shape? How old are you?

Why am I asking these questions? Because if you're 5'2" and not similarly shaped, you're never going to have Angelina Jolie's body. I happen to think

Kelly Ripa has an amazing body. I would love to have her arms. I'm also close to six feet tall and have to be realistic about what my muscles look like.

Now for a few names you might not recognize: Ray Kybartas, Karen Voight, Gunnar Peterson, Bob Greene...Ringing any bells? These are the fitness gurus who cater to stars such as Madonna, Brooke Burke, Heidi Klum and many, many others.

I harbor a deep appreciation for these trainers and fitness experts because they help people live more healthfully by promoting good nutrition and exercise as a way of life, but I can't afford to hire these trainers to work out with me on a semi-weekly basis. I can't afford a nanny, a nutritionist or a world-class chef, either. Can you?

More importantly, are you being paid to look perfect because your face and body sell movies, magazines, clothes and makeup? Or are you an accountant, lawyer, teacher, student, salesperson, businessperson or stay-at-home mom? When you download pictures of yourself, do you have the ability to shave off ten to fifteen pounds, correct pimples and draw in muscle tone with a click of a mouse?

I hope I'm driving home an important point here: we are not on an even playing field with celebrities, and while it's fine to want to emulate them, don't let it become an unhealthy obsession. In other words…

Stop comparing yourself to others!

Focusing your attention on someone else detracts from the attention you should be giving yourself. Not everyone is built like a supermodel. Not everyone has a reality TV show. Like so many other women, you probably have a very long list of tasks each day, and if your household is like mine, the only person around to do them is you. With your busy day in mind, I say start off with baby steps.

First of all, stop blaming yourself. It's important to understand how you got here, so look back and learn from it. There's no point in looking back to blame yourself. Look back only to understand what got you here so that you can get to work correcting it.

Be loving and kind and begin to care for yourself on every level, including food. Set realistic goals for yourself. How much weight do you need to lose?

Attack these pounds in increments of ten. Reaching small goals is more attainable than reaching large ones, and getting that first ten pounds off is incredibly motivating.

After all, if you're devouring this chapter, it's no doubt because you've had a baby, or two or three, and maybe you're having trouble shedding your baby weight. Maybe you're just jealous of women you see who seem to regain their figures with ease, especially all those celebrities staring at you from the pages of magazines while you're standing in the grocery store check-out line. Trust me. This is all part of…

The wonderful world of motherhood!

Motherhood is wonderful, but it does take a toll. Sleep deprivation aside, let's talk about the realities of your body post-baby. Did you step on the scale and find that giving birth to that munchkin didn't erase the pounds you gained while incubating your little bundle of joy? Has it been a week or so since you gave birth, yet you still look four months pregnant? If you had a C-section, do you have to be lowered onto the toilet to tinkle?

Who knew that a C-section was a "major" surgery and that you utilize your abdominal muscles for, oh, just about everything? Walking, sleeping, sitting, lying down, picking up your new baby, holding your other children (if you have any), laughing, sneezing...if you can name it, you probably need abdominal muscles to do it.

If you had a "regular" childbirth, you're no doubt dealing with a whole other realm of post-baby pains, but I wouldn't know much about that, having had two C-sections.

At this point, the point at which you're standing on the scale, you're probably praying for a miracle while asking yourself some key questions: how much did I gain? What about my gigantic new post-baby breasts? Don't they weigh five pounds each? How did that Celebrity Mommy lose her weight anyway? Nursing, right? Doesn't nursing melt fat?

This is the part of new motherhood that nobody warned you about, the part where you're standing in line at the grocery store staring at trash magazines wondering how semi-celeb is on the cover in a bikini just months after having a baby. Some new moms are inspired; other new moms want to gag.

Whichever category you fit into, be patient with yourself. And get real. Remember, you don't have the nanny, the trainer, the nutritionist, or the chef on staff. Put the trash magazine down and look in the mirror. Whom do YOU want to look like? If you must use a celeb as motivation, pick one who closely resembles your own body structure and is close to your age.

What celebrity did I channel when I was finally ready to lose the weight for once and for all?

Myself. I took an old picture of myself, from a time when I was exuberantly happy and healthy, and taped it to my mirror and fridge. As the weight came off, I was closer and closer to looking like that old picture until finally I stopped looking at it, because I was looking right at her in the mirror.

Forget celebumom. Celebuyou.

Key points in this chapter:

- Stop comparing yourself to others.

- Get real – it took you nine months to grow your beautiful baby. You're not going to – you're not even supposed to – look "normal" again for some time.

- Celebrate yourself – no one else on the planet could have delivered the child you now love more than life itself.

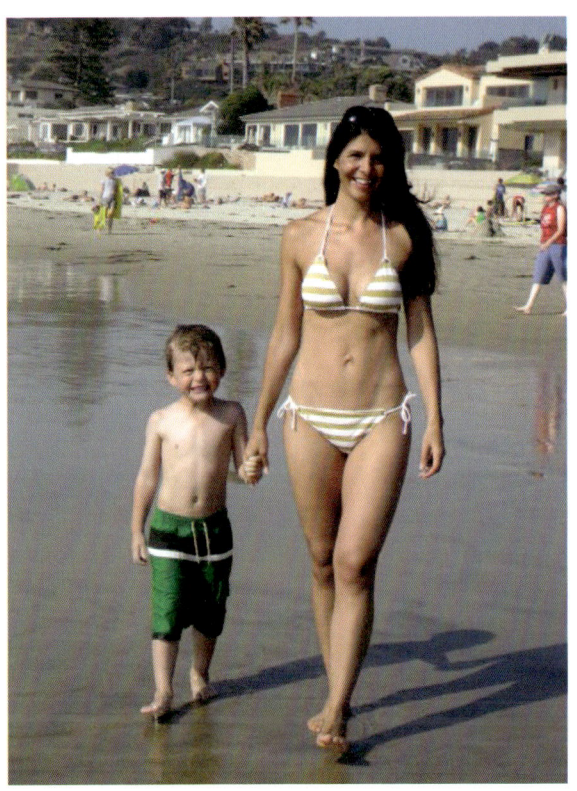

Original photo of Tania and her son

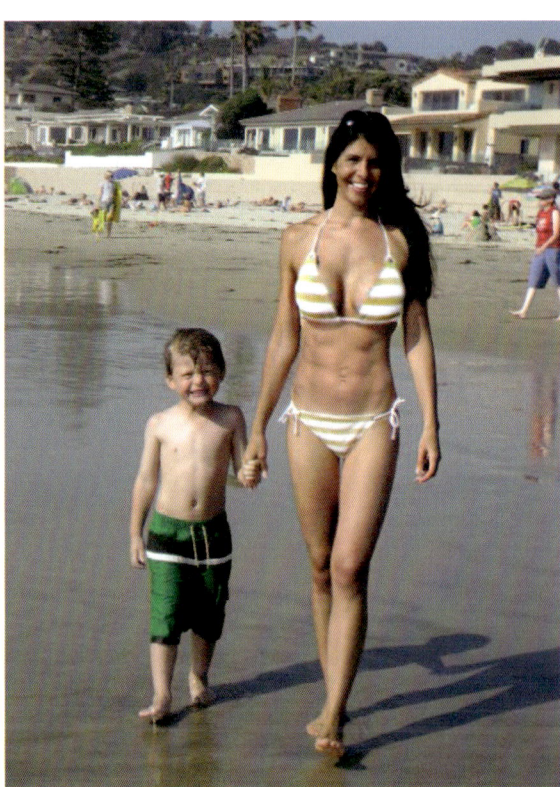

Same photo digitally enhanced with Photoshop

Section 2 :

Tip the Scale in Your Favor

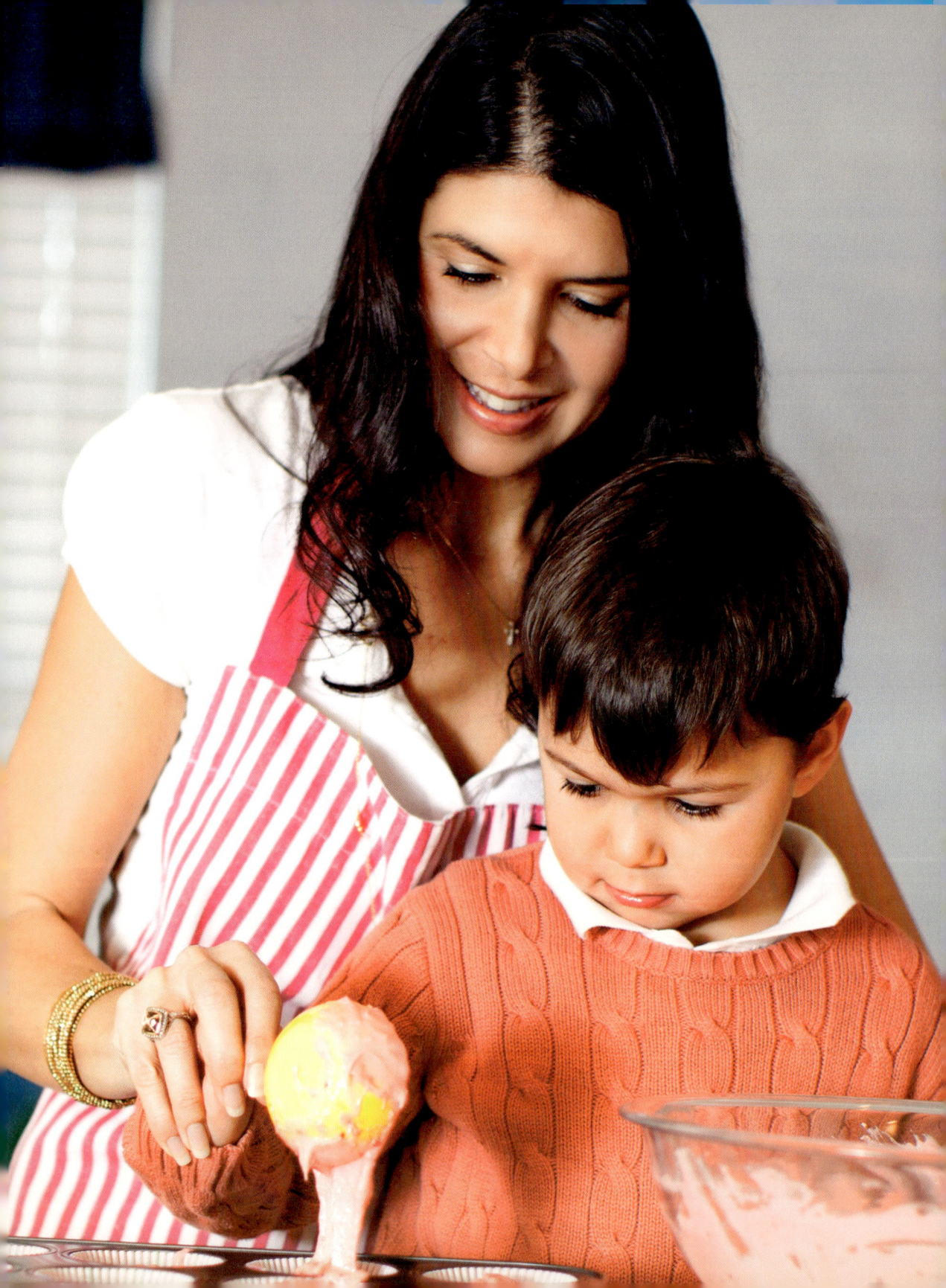

Chapter 4 :

Eliminate the "Frenemies"

I say "eliminate" in the kindest way possible and obviously I'm not being literal, but the quickest way to get started and hold yourself accountable is by telling ALL the people in your camp that you've made a decision to get healthy.

Frequently this goes well, but sometimes the people in your life are not supportive. Sometimes they're scared of change or unhappy with their own lifestyles. These people question your motives and methods, they become negative naysayers, and they dig at you about your choices and undermine your goals. Get rid of them! At least until you're halfway to your goal and are comfortable standing up for yourself.

Unfortunately, I've encountered this a few times from people who were friends, some overweight, some not. Their own feelings of inadequacy led them to criticize my goals and achievements. Here's a sprinkling of typical comments I heard from those "frenemies" as I began to lose weight:

"Aren't you starving?"

"I'm going to eat food that tastes good; how's your cardboard?"

"OMG, you look so UNHEALTHY! Are you anorexic?" (I must admit, this is my personal favorite.)

"Get real, sister," I always wanted to say. "I've lost EIGHT FREAKING POUNDS and have FORTY to go!"

Ditch these negative naysayers for the time being, or at least refuse to banter with them about your goals. Instead,

Gather support from your inner circle

You need all the support and accountability you can get, because it's EASY to backslide and give in to temptation. To quote my friend Clint Herzog, you want people in your camp who pass the "mom test."

What is the "mom test"? Simple. When you have great news, or bad news, or you've made a decision, or you just want to talk, who do you call? You call the people who are always in your corner and are more excited about your news than even YOU are. These people are always supportive of you, no matter what news you're breaking.

Let's face it. For some people, their mother does NOT fill this role, but you catch my drift. There are people in your life who do fill this role, and these are the individuals you want to support you in your new decision to start eating and living healthfully.

Now that we've covered the mom test, let's address and engage your partner if you have one. Many, many people on the road to weight loss have told me they often don't have support within their own households. This is very sad. It is unbelievably hard to lose weight when the person on the couch next to you is pounding soda, chips or chocolate and you're eating carrot sticks.

I'm not saying they need to change their lifestyle with you, but they do need to be supportive of your decision to commit to good health. Give them bonus points if they join you on your journey, but think twice if they actively undermine you.

My best experience in this regard happened with my friend Scarlett in Georgia. She and I had worked at the same property management company and together we made the decision to lose weight. We ate healthfully and made a daily commitment to exercise, walking our community two to four miles almost every day for four months. The weight came off rapidly for both of us. It was SO motivating to have each other for accountability, companionship and support!

I guess what I'm really saying is to surround yourself with people who are sensitive to the goals you are trying to reach. After all, how can you possibly stick to your guns when your roommate or partner is urging you to join them for "just one" donut? Hopefully you'll have support in this important endeavor. But don't forget,

It took time to get here

Think about it. How much TIME did it take you to get this big? How much TIME did you spend eating poorly and sitting on the couch? How much TIME do you have to LIVE if you continue this lifestyle? Finally, how much TIME are you willing to invest to make yourself healthy?

I use the word "invest" because this decision IS an investment. It's an investment in your future that will pay off big time by eliminating certain very significant health dangers that accompany obesity.

Personally, it took me nine months to gain just my baby weight, so there was no way it was going to evaporate in thirty days. I gave myself a goal of one year to eliminate my spare tires, and I made it in much less time than that. But one reason this worked was that I remembered to do the following…
Carve out time for yourself

TIME again. Yes, time for yourself must be SCHEDULED. Otherwise, it's very unlikely you'll get any, because good intentions are not enough. You have to have a plan, and you NEED to carve out a little time every day to get moving and do something healthy for yourself.

From a food perspective, it does take a little time to prepare a fresh, healthy omelet with all egg whites, fresh veggies and just a smidge of cheese. I admit it; the drive-thru IS easier. But when you give in to the drive-thru, you're ordering yourself a fat bomb, and weight loss does not come in a drive-thru bag. Haven't we already covered that?

Key points in this chapter:

- Lose your frenemies.

- Don't share your weight-loss news with everyone in your life, just the people who pass your "mom test" and are in your camp.

- Good intentions are not enough. Take the TIME to exercise and cook healthfully, and give yourself time to lose your excess weight for good.

- Fast = FAT!

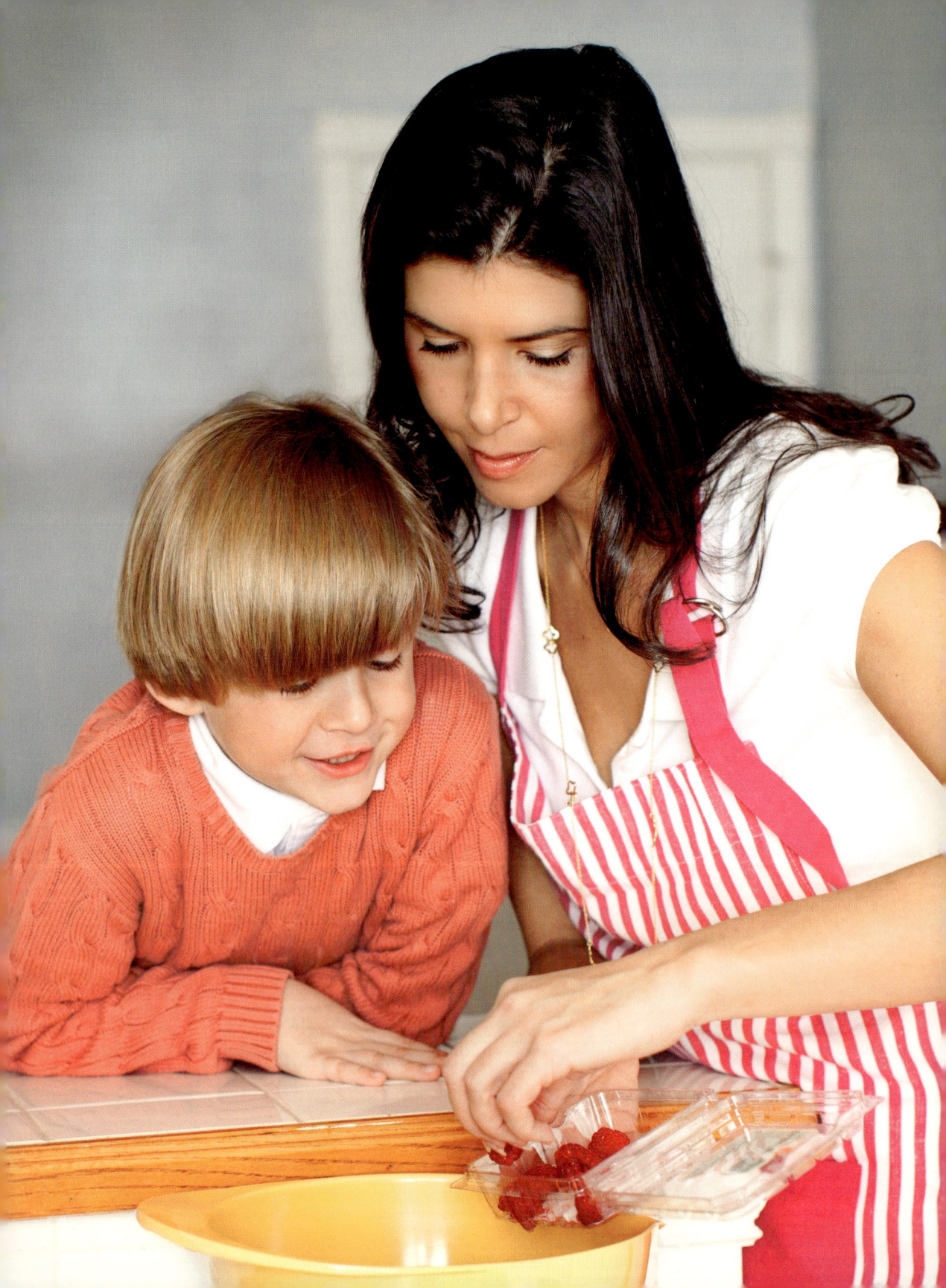

Chapter 5:

The Science of "Skinny"

(with an excerpt from fitness expert Marc Zalmanoff)

In this chapter, I want you to ask yourself four questions:

1. Do you want to be skinny?

2. Do you want to be healthy?

3. Do you want to be fit?

4. Do you want to look good?

Answer these questions honestly and see the graph below. Your goal should be to land in the middle where the three circles overlap. The only tools you need to get there are the foods you eat plus the amount you exercise.

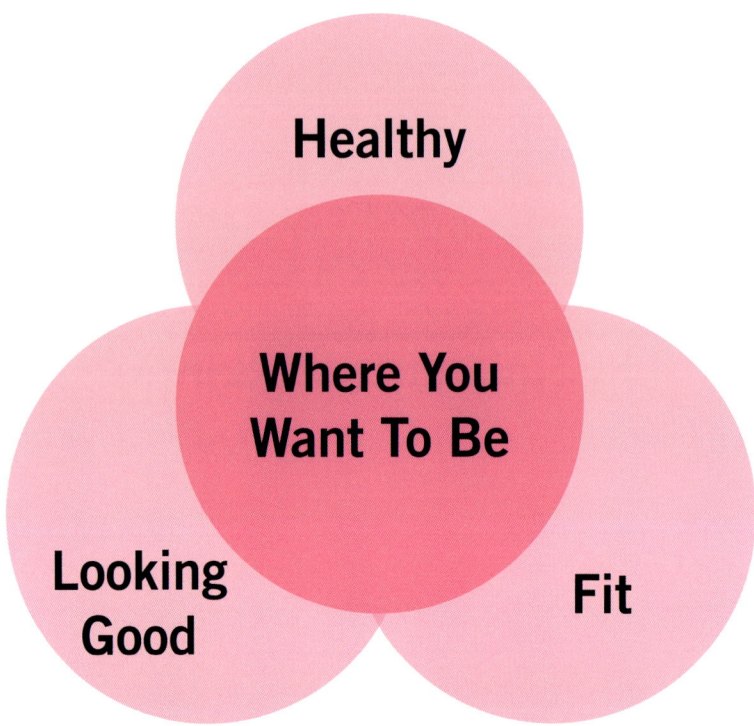

Let's address each circle one by one.

The first circle is "Healthy." Healthy is good, but there is such a thing as trying to be too healthy. Some people in this category go overboard on the all-naturals, the omegas, the granolas and the healthy fats. When you're too focused on this category, you might be overloading on fats and not eating lean enough.

What do I mean? As an example, let's break down the nutrition facts of granola. You have nuts, raisins and grains covered in sugar or honey and dried out in the sun. These are sugar and fat bombs, my friends! Granted, these are "healthy" fats, but why not skip the sugar and go for whole roasted almonds instead? A certain amount of Omegas ARE necessary to maintain your shiny hair and strong bones and nails, but neither man nor woman can survive on trail mix alone!

The next circle is "Looking Good." The danger of focusing solely on this circle is that you're eating TOO lean, thereby depleting your body of those essential fats we discussed in the previous paragraph. Is it your goal to look like a competitive bodybuilder? Probably not.

People in this category tend to go overboard on nutrition bars, shakes and manufactured foods. What they seldom realize is that the toxins that are pumped into their systems from the energy drinks and fabricated "nutrition" bars would make your head spin! What the heck is Isomalto-oligosaccharide anyway? Have you heard of it? Does it sound like you should be eating it? Do yourself a favor and grab an apple!

Finally, our last circle is "Fit." Are you a cardio freak? Do you tailor your entire life around the classes at your gym or have more than one membership? Do you "club hop" so you can utilize the kid's club for four hours a day instead of the typical two? Does your family complain about how much you're away doing things for your body and that you're not spending enough time with them? Do you lift weights every single day for hours or max out at the gym on a weekly basis?

The end result of becoming a gym rat is that you either burn out or you ruin your joints and muscles, making yourself so sore you begin to associate pain with exercise, not to mention the wear and tear on your family because you're never home.

Don't just take my word for it. For this chapter, I did in fact consult with an expert. My close friend Marc Zalmanoff, of Stay Young Fitness in Frisco, Texas, has some pointers and tips to get you and your body in "the middle zone" of these three circles. Here is what he has to say…

From an expert…

Probably the hardest aspect of weight loss for most people is figuring out where to start. In my opinion, the actual starting point is in your head. You have to make up your mind that being fit, living healthier and taking better care of yourself is a priority. We all lead busy lives, we all have reasons why we can't work out, and we can all find a million other things that need to be done instead of productively burning some calories.

But that is precisely the problem with so many people: we put everyone else's needs ahead of our own…our spouses, our parents, our children, our bosses, our co-workers. In the process, we completely neglect ourselves. I believe most of us are people pleasers by nature, but we cannot be there to support the ones we love if we do not take care of ourselves first.

I'm here to tell you that you are worth it. You are worth the time, you are worth the effort and you deserve a happy, healthy life. I'm a firm believer that everything in life happens for a reason. These reasons may not always be clear at the present time, but eventually they are revealed. There's a reason you are reading this book right now and there's a reason it's this message you are hearing.

I can't tell you how many times I've heard "I wish" from a client, as in "I wish I'd worked out twenty years ago" or "I wish I'd changed my habits before I developed heart disease" or "I wish I'd listened to my instinct and done something when it was time for bigger pants!"

Sometimes the road ahead seems overwhelming, but when the risk it takes to remain the same is more painful than the risk to change, that is when you will truly embrace the journey ahead.

Please let that resonate for a minute. Too many people unnecessarily live in pain, with stomachaches and joint pains, heartburn and sleep apnea, headaches and diabetes, most of which can be prevented if we choose to deliberately make healthy choices in our lives. So now you have to dig deep, figure out what truly motivates you, and get moving! And the first thing you'll need to do is…

Exercise!

Ah, the part you've been waiting for…or dreading.

Here's a cheesy yet insightful cliché to get you going: A journey of a thousand miles begins with the first step.

Perhaps you've heard that a time or two? It certainly rings true in this instance. The first step of any good exercise program is setting forth a plan. Now, everyone's plan is different, and much like your goals in general, your plan has to be realistic to your lifestyle, so let's start with some general guidelines. I love acronyms, so we will now apply the F.I.T.T. principle, which consists of the following:

- Frequency, or how often you exercise. The surgeon general says you should exercise most days of the week. My recommendation is a minimum of four times per week, more if possible.

- Intensity, or how hard you work during exercise. This varies greatly with what you are doing and where your fitness level currently resides. My theory has always been to push yourself. At some point, you must step out of your comfort zone, face your fears head on and attack your workouts like a spider monkey. This may not always be the greatest feeling during your workouts, but you will feel fantastic afterwards! Pushing yourself brings a sense of accomplishment that very little else can match. No, I'm not suggesting you become the cardio freak at the gym. Moderation in all things…including moderation.

- Time, or how long you exercise. This will often come down to the time you have available. Ideally, forty-five to sixty minutes is ample time to get a complete workout done, regardless of what you are trying to accomplish that day.

- Type, or what type of activity you're doing. This is all about personal preference. You must find something that appeals to you. If running reminds you of high school gym class, horrible green shorts and doing laps because someone was late to class, then it may not be for you. The best exercise is something you will enjoy (at least a little bit, anyway) so that you are motivated to do more. If you like what you're doing, your odds of success are much greater.

With all that said, the appendix at the back of the book offers an easy-to-follow gym fitness plan to get you started on a successful path. Adhere to these guidelines for the next three months, and I know you will be a better, healthier person. In the meantime, take advantage of what I like to call…

Marc's and Tania's Tips for Success

As if dealing with us one at a time weren't enough, Tania and I have teamed up to offer some life-changing tips to help you be successful in your health and wellness journey. We know that the best-laid plans can be disrupted by the unforeseen, but having a plan in the first place is, we believe, critical to long-term success. Since the nutrition realm is so critical to sustained weight loss, here are some tips to remember when it comes to dieting:

- Drink water while you eat. Not only will this slow down your actual eating process, the water will make you feel full faster, which means you will eat less.

- Use small plates and utensils, such as your kids' unbreakable plastic monkey plates and even their Elmo spoons. This allows you to still fill your plate up, but with a normal portion size. The smaller utensils force you to take smaller bites and slow down while you're eating.

- Put your fork down between bites. Many of us scarf our food down without taking a breath, devouring everything in sight before our bodies can catch up. Often, our stomachs become full but our brains don't yet know it. By slowing down, you can get your mind and body to connect at the same time and avoid that "UGH" feeling you get from eating too much too fast.

- Put half your meal in a to-go box. If you're dining out, get a box and immediately put half your meal in there before you start eating. This will still allow you to clean your plate but will limit you to a more reasonable amount of food.

- Plan ahead. Again, if you're eating out, check the menu online before you arrive. Make a healthy decision ahead of time and don't even look at the menu.

- Talk. Not with your mouth full, of course, but if you have someone to talk to while you're eating, it will slow you down, which will produce the same effect as putting your fork down between bites.

- Pour salt on it. This is one of our all-time favorites, and no, we're not suggesting you increase your salt intake. Instead, when you're done eating, or know you should be, grab the nearest salt shaker and literally DUMP salt all over your plate. It's very easy to keep picking at a dish after you know you should be done, but with a plethora of salt all over it, it probably won't be as appetizing anymore.

Now, here are some tips to consider in the fitness realm:

Eliminate "I can't" from your vocabulary. Forbid yourself to use that phrase. Henry Ford once said, "Whether you think you can or you can't, you're right." Believe in yourself, and believe that almost anything is possible when you set your mind to it.

We'll say it again...Find something you truly enjoy. Not every workout will be fun and games and you won't always WANT to get up and go, but finding activities that provide some inherent pleasure will go a long way towards keeping you motivated. Whether it's running, cycling, weightlifting, aerobic classes, boot camp, or a combination of them all, find something you love and make it part of your routine.

If you are trying to lose weight, keep the biggest article of clothing you have. As the pounds begin to drop, get rid of the sizes you no longer need, but keep one item as a reminder of where you were. On the reverse side of things, dig out that pair of jeans you stored away in the recesses of your mind and closet, the ones you told yourself you'd probably never fit into again, and pull them out. Hang them somewhere prominent and tell yourself every day that you WILL wear them proudly again! Tania's favorite saying, "the only thing better than new clothes, is old clothes that fit again" is so true!

Make exercise a part of your everyday routine. Find the time that works best for you and put it on your schedule. You are more likely to stay consistent when the thought process is "It's time to go work out now" instead of "I hope I make it to the gym today."

Your efforts to have a more fit, healthier body should not go without reward. We believe it is human nature to want a little pat on the back for a job well done. It's a great feeling to see the belt slip another notch, to notice a muscle we never had before, or to accomplish a task not previously possible. The problem is, we human beings tend to celebrate everything with food, which completely defeats the purpose behind the sweat and labored breathing of working out.

Here a few ways to reward yourself without filling up your belly:

- Go shopping. A changing body often means you need new clothes. Properly fitting clothes can make you feel more confident and are a great reflection of your hard work.

- Go to the movies. Movies are a great little treat to escape reality and relax. Needless to say, don't get the ten-gallon tub of popcorn while you're there.

- Try a new activity. With newfound fitness can come newfound abilities (or at least the willingness to try). Hiking, biking and indoor rock climbing can be fun recreational activities to explore. If you like them enough, they can even become part of your fitness routine.

- Get a massage. This is by FAR our favorite! There's nothing like lying there doing nothing while being pampered. If you are working out on a regular basis, massage is a great tool as it can help alleviate soreness and muscle imbalance. Plus, it just plain feels good, and besides…

Now is the time!

There really is no time like the present to take action. When we want something in life, I mean REALLY want something, we waste no time in getting started, and your health should be no exception. If you've made up your mind that a happier, healthier you is in your future, take action NOW!

Don't wait until Monday, or the first of the month, or until after your birthday, or the week after your anniversary, or until you've returned from that vacation that's just "impossible" to eat healthy on. Start NOW! In fact, take a break from reading this and do a set of pushups to warm yourself up.

Back so soon, or didn't you do it? Give yourself a quick analysis. Where are you right now? Are you losing weight and becoming a healthier individual, or are you like so many who are slowly gaining weight or merely maintaining a weight they're unhappy with in an unhealthy lifestyle?

Just remember, if you do what you've always done, you'll get what you've always had. Einstein once said the definition of insanity is doing the same thing over and over again and expecting a different result. You must choose a different path to achieve the great things you are capable of achieving. Use the tools, tips and tricks outlined in this book and start your journey TODAY!

Key points in this chapter:

- Does your weight loss goal land you in the middle where the three circles overlap?

- Do you believe you're worth the effort to make necessary changes?

- Remember, moderation in all things…including moderation.

- Follow our nutrition and exercise tips to increase your chances of success.

- Don't turn to food as a reward for reaching goals.

- Begin today to take action to be healthier, happier and more fit.

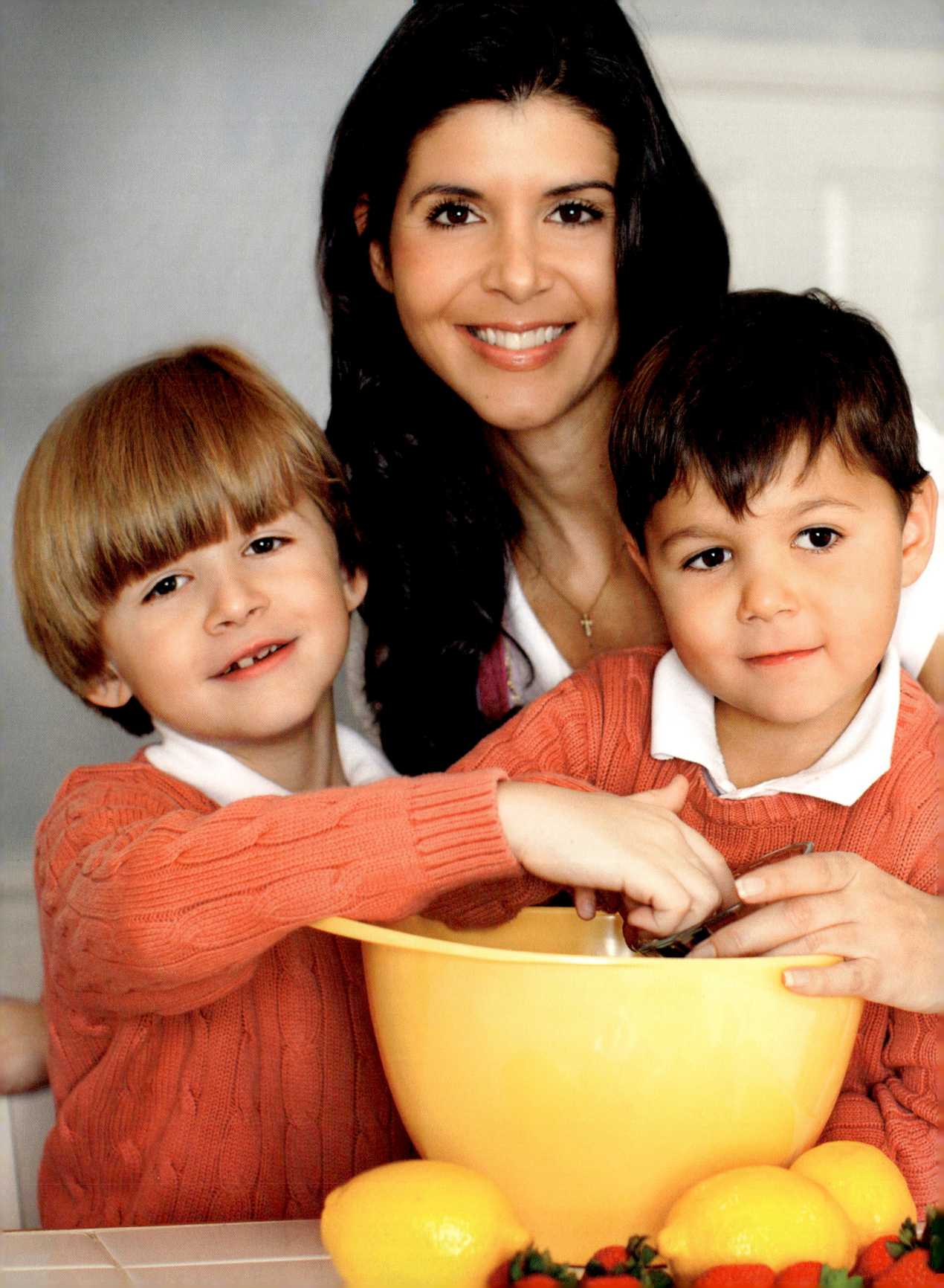

Chapter 6:

Nutrition In Your Kitchen

So here we are. You've realized you need to change a few things, but you aren't certain where to start. Don't let yourself get overwhelmed with details and "to do" lists. Just start in the most logical place you can think of.

For me, that's the grocery store. Unless you grow a lot of your own food, this is where your nutrition is going to come from. Having learned the hard way how to properly approach a grocery store, I'd like to share with you my two musts: you must begin on a full stomach, and you must, if possible, go on Saturday morning. A full stomach prevents you from making impulsive low blood sugar decisions, and Saturday mornings work because the market is usually a ghost town. But before you leave home, make an effort to…

Understand your choices

You may shop in the same store week after week, or you may hit whatever store is on your errand route on any given day. Either way, pay attention to the way the store is laid out. Typically, breads, cakes and "convenience" foods are easy to get to, right up front, and the first thing you see and smell. Enticing, eh?

Keep on moving past those demons of despair to the "fresh" sections and the outer walls of your market. This is where you'll find your veggies, fruits, meats, seafood, dairy and most unprocessed foods.

When entering the aisles of your store, notice too that the fatty and unhealthy choices are typically right at eye level. Look to the bottom and top of the shelves for your healthier options. For example, my favorite flax seed granola cereal is always on the very tiptop of the shelf.

But before you go to the grocery store, make sure you know what you're going for. Otherwise, you run the risk of filling your cart with things you believe are healthy but in reality are just cleverly packaged to fool you.

This means you need to prepare a menu and figure out what you already have on hand. In other words, before you can shop, you need a list of what you DON'T have in your cupboard. Before you can create that list, you need to...

Check out your pantry

My absolute staples? Shockingly, I have only a few. These include egg whites, tomatoes, low fat cheese, salsa, ketchup, oatmeal, Greek yogurt, Nature's Path granola cereal, reduced-fat peanut butter, smoked almonds, whole wheat bread and tortillas, black beans, fresh boneless, skinless chicken, salad mixes, and finally, tremendous amounts of fruits and vegetables.

I also keep Truvia and Splenda on hand for sweetening because Truvia is all natural and has zero calories and Splenda is fabulous for baking. I Can't Believe It's Not Butter Light is also a favorite because it maintains a buttery flavor, is great for baking, and is significantly lower in fat than the real deal.

These staples should be kept on hand and restocked when they get low. If you don't have a magnetic notepad on your fridge on which to keep a list of needed items, get one. It's a lifesaver, and as the kids grow, they can start scribbling down items, too.

I also keep bulk foods like grains – think barley, brown rice, etc. –on hand in jars or bags. When I need them, I've got them. This frees up my grocery cart for the fresh fruits, vegetables and dairy items that don't keep so well.

All told, the following items are essential to a well-stocked pantry. Buy them at the store and eat them at home, and you'll be well on your way to a happier, healthier you.

Vegetables

asparagus
beets
broccoli
brussels sprouts
cabbage
collards
cauliflower
celery
cucumber
eggplant
greens
 (baby or dark leafy)
garlic
jicama
kale
mushrooms
onions
peppers
scallions
spinach
sprouts
squash
sweet potatoes
tomatoes
zucchini

Fruits

apples
apricots
avocado
berries
cherries
citrus
olives
peaches
pears
plums
tropical fruits

Meats, Poultry and Fish

lean ground beef
flank steak
tenderloin
lean ham
white meat chicken
white meat turkey
white tuna

cod
crab
orange roughy
salmon
shrimp
snapper
tuna

Dairy

low-fat milk
low-fat cheese
low-fat cottage cheese
low-fat or fat-free
 Greek yogurt
low-fat or fat-free
 cream cheese
low-fat or fat-free
 sour cream
low-fat or fat-free plain
 or flavored yogurt
low-fat ice cream and
 treats (in moderation!)

Grains

barley
brown rice
buckwheat
corn
couscous
kasha
millet
oats
quinoa
rice
rye
spelt

This is a lot of food. A lot of beautiful, healthy food. Now that you've purchased it, you need to get it home and put it away. Do you have a place for everything? As needed, think it through and take the time to…

Organize your kitchen

Before we get to the all-important Simply Sinless recipes that make this cookbook so unique, it's important to take a good hard look at your kitchen and get it ready for the new lifestyle you're about to embark on. Organize it, reorganize it, or call in the carpenters and start from scratch. Just get it ready. What do I mean?

Move the skillets, saucepans and bakeware to a cupboard you can easily access. The same goes for your spices, measuring cups and spoons. Remember, if it's too difficult to reach your muffin pan, you'll end up in a coffee house ordering a 500-calorie fat bomb you could have made lighter – and more economically – at home.

Think about the rooms in your house in a "big picture" sort of way. You have a formal dining area and it looks beautiful, but chances are, you only sit there for Easter, Thanksgiving and Christmas dinners. The remainder of the year, you're in the breakfast nook with the small, comfortably crowded table and all of your family around you. Why? It's comfortable and feels like home. Chances are, when you're done with Thanksgiving meals, you retire to THIS table for dessert.

Same goes for your beautiful formal living room. Most of the time, aren't you more inclined to spend time in the comfy den with the raggedy sofa, smoldering fireplace and big screen TV?

Apply the same principle to your kitchen. If you have bright fluorescent lighting, soften it. If you have cookbooks that slam closed, buy a cookbook stand. If you have room to sit but nothing to sit on, grab a stool at your favorite second-hand store.

Bottom line, make your kitchen comfy and you'll ENJOY being in there! By extension, if you enjoy being in there, you're far more likely to use the recipes in this book. Which brings me to…

The reasons for the recipes

At long last, we're moving into the part of the book that probably reflects why you bought it in the first place. I've chosen the following recipes carefully, which leads me to a quick and insightful story. One recent day, my lovely boyfriend asked "T, why are you putting Mexican recipes in this book? Isn't this a health food cookbook? Isn't Mexican food counterproductive?"

My answer to this is simple: I don't make "health food." I'm taking recipes I love and making them healthier and hopefully keeping you out of the drive-thru. I've learned that I CAN look like a body builder if I eat only tuna, chicken, boiled eggs and low starch carbs. I can also attest to the fact that I WILL end up face down in a box of Little Debbies if I try to maintain this eating regimen for more than a week.

Bottom line, if it doesn't taste good, you aren't going to eat it, any more than I am. But that doesn't mean it has to be loaded with fat, butter and cream. What it means, once again, is moderation. So let's get ready to cook your way to a healthier, leaner you.

Section 3 :

Recipes for Change

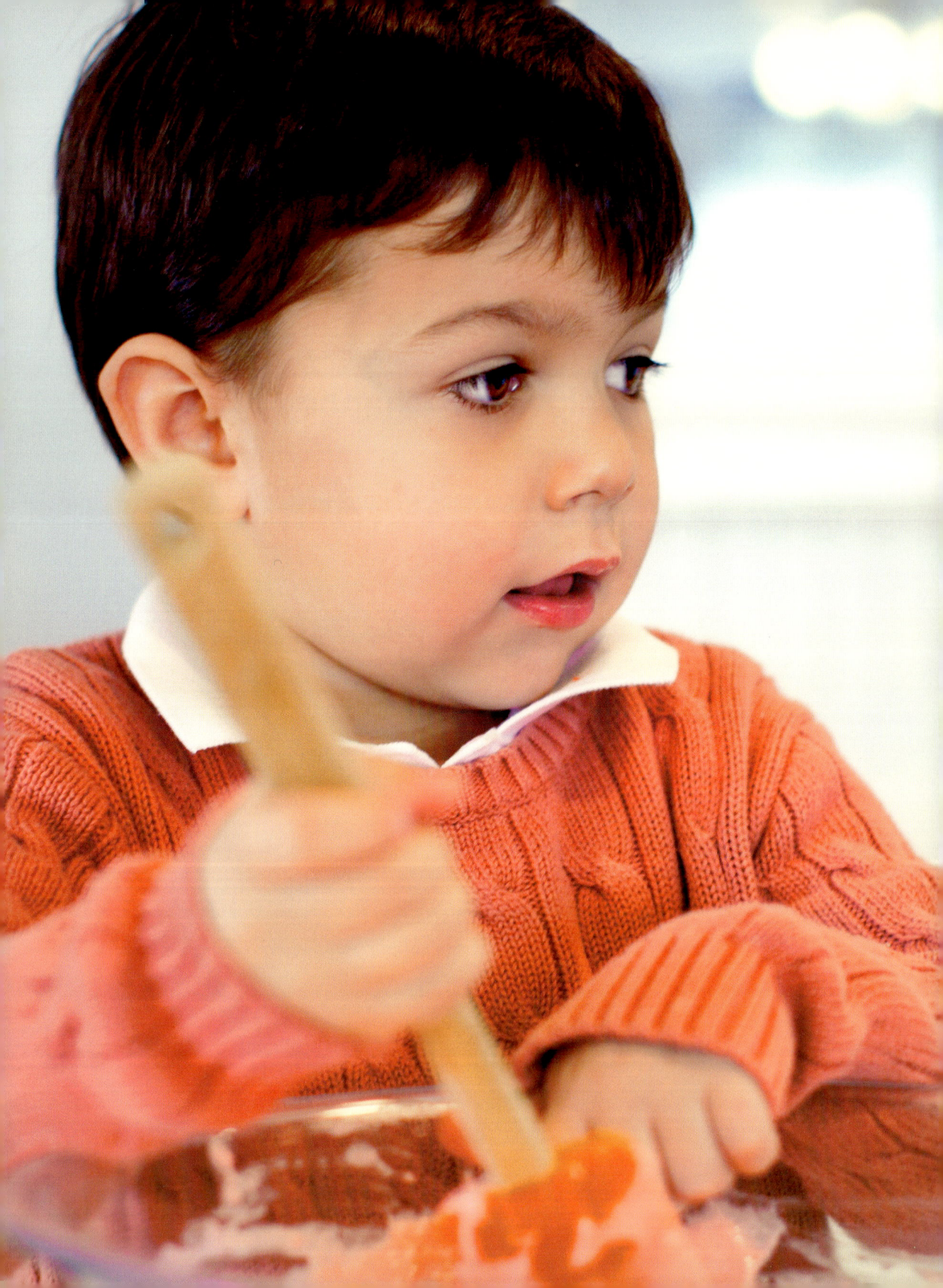

Chapter 7:

Simply Sinless Breakfasts

The recipes that follow are tried and true. They're also relatively easy, but if you're short on time, head for the ones that contain "Simply Sinless" in the title. Each of these Simply Sinless recipes contains fewer than ten ingredients and takes the least time to prepare.

And are they ever delicious…

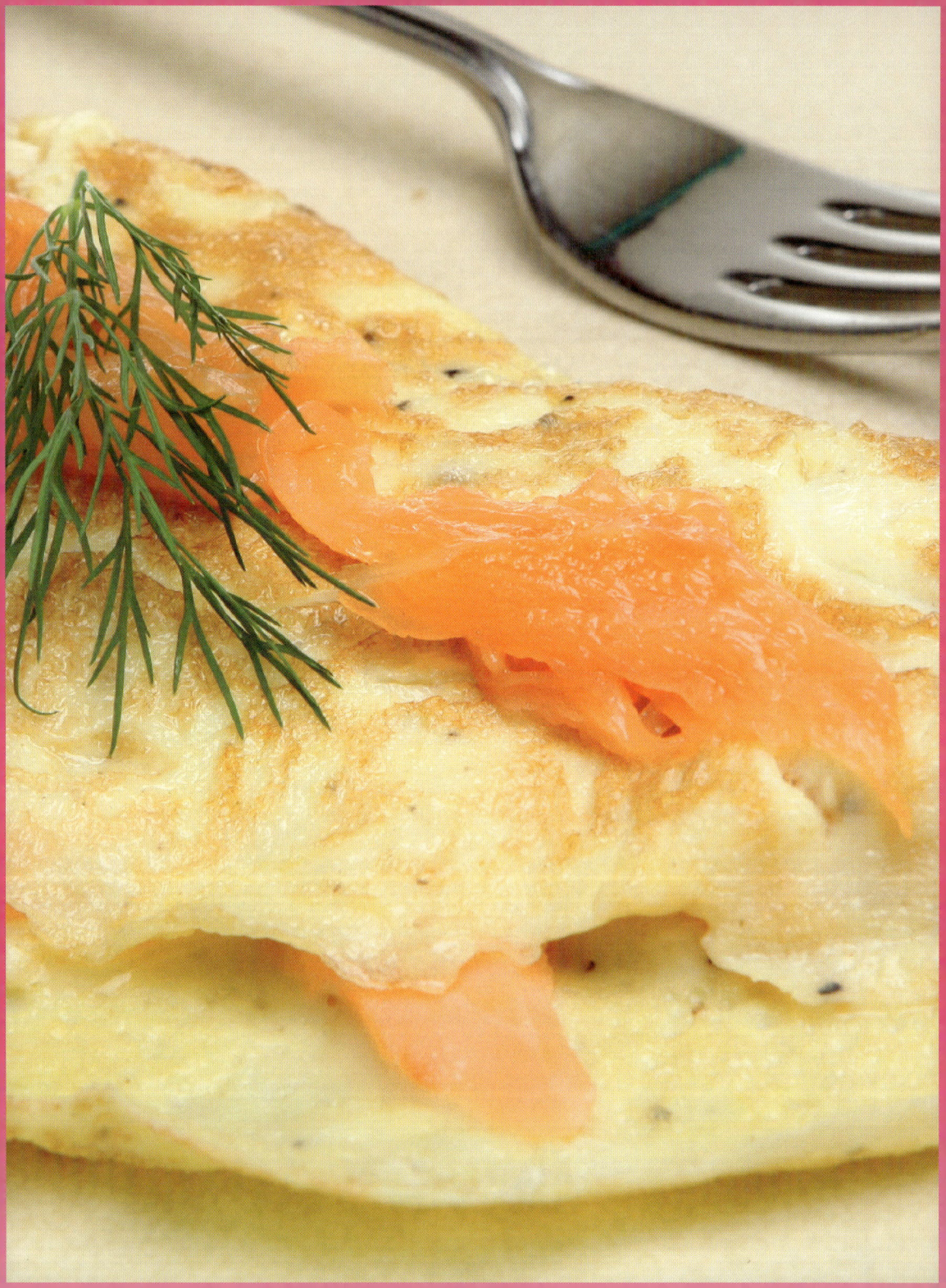

Simply Sinless Smoked Salmon & Cream Cheese Omelet

INGREDIENTS

1 cup egg whites
4 teaspoons nonfat or light cream cheese
1 ounce smoked salmon
Fat-free cooking spray, olive oil flavor
Sea salt
Cracked black pepper
Smidge of olive oil

DIRECTIONS

1. Coat nonstick skillet with fat-free cooking spray and add a smidge of olive oil. Whisk together egg whites, cream cheese, salt and pepper and pour into prepared skillet. Cook over medium to high heat, gently moving the mixture around as it cooks.

2. When eggs are almost finished cooking, add the salmon to the top of the eggs and cover for 30 seconds to a minute. Remove lid, add a little more salt and pepper, slide omelet onto plate, fold in half, and serve with fresh fruit or whole wheat toast.

Serves 2.

Simply Sinless Spicy Scramble

INGREDIENTS

3 egg whites (or 2 egg whites and 1 egg, depending on taste preference)
¼ cup canned black beans, drained and rinsed
2 tablespoons hot salsa
2 tablespoons reduced-fat cheddar cheese
Sea salt
Cracked black pepper
1 whole grain tortilla

DIRECTIONS

1. Coat nonstick skillet with fat-free cooking spray and place on medium heat.

2. Scramble all ingredients together, adding salt and pepper to taste.

3. Warm the whole grain tortilla and fill with the spicy scramble or serve on the side.

Serves 1, but feel free to multiply recipe as needed for more servings.

Beautiful Brunch Ham Strata

INGREDIENTS

4   pieces whole grain bread

2   cups sliced mushrooms

1/3 cup chopped red bell pepper

1/3 cup minced red onion

5   slices lean ham
       (sliced thin for sandwiches is best)

4   cups baby spinach

1 1/2 cups egg whites

1   cup skim milk

3   tablespoons reduced-fat Parmesan
       Nonstick cooking spray
       Salt
       Black pepper

DIRECTIONS

1. Toast whole grain bread and lightly spray bottom of a small baking dish with nonstick cooking spray. Place the four slices of toasted bread on the bottom of the baking dish.

2. Lightly spray a large skillet with nonstick cooking spray and add the mushrooms, pepper and minced red onion and sauté for 5 minutes.

3. Add the baby spinach and lean ham and sauté for 1 minute.

4. In a bowl, combine the egg whites and skim milk and stir until well blended. Pour over bread and top with sautéed veggies and ham.

5. Sprinkle the three tablespoons of reduced-fat Parmesan over the top of the veggies and season with salt and pepper to taste.

6. Bake at 450 degrees for about 15 minutes or until egg is fully cooked. Serve hot and enjoy!

Serves 6-8.

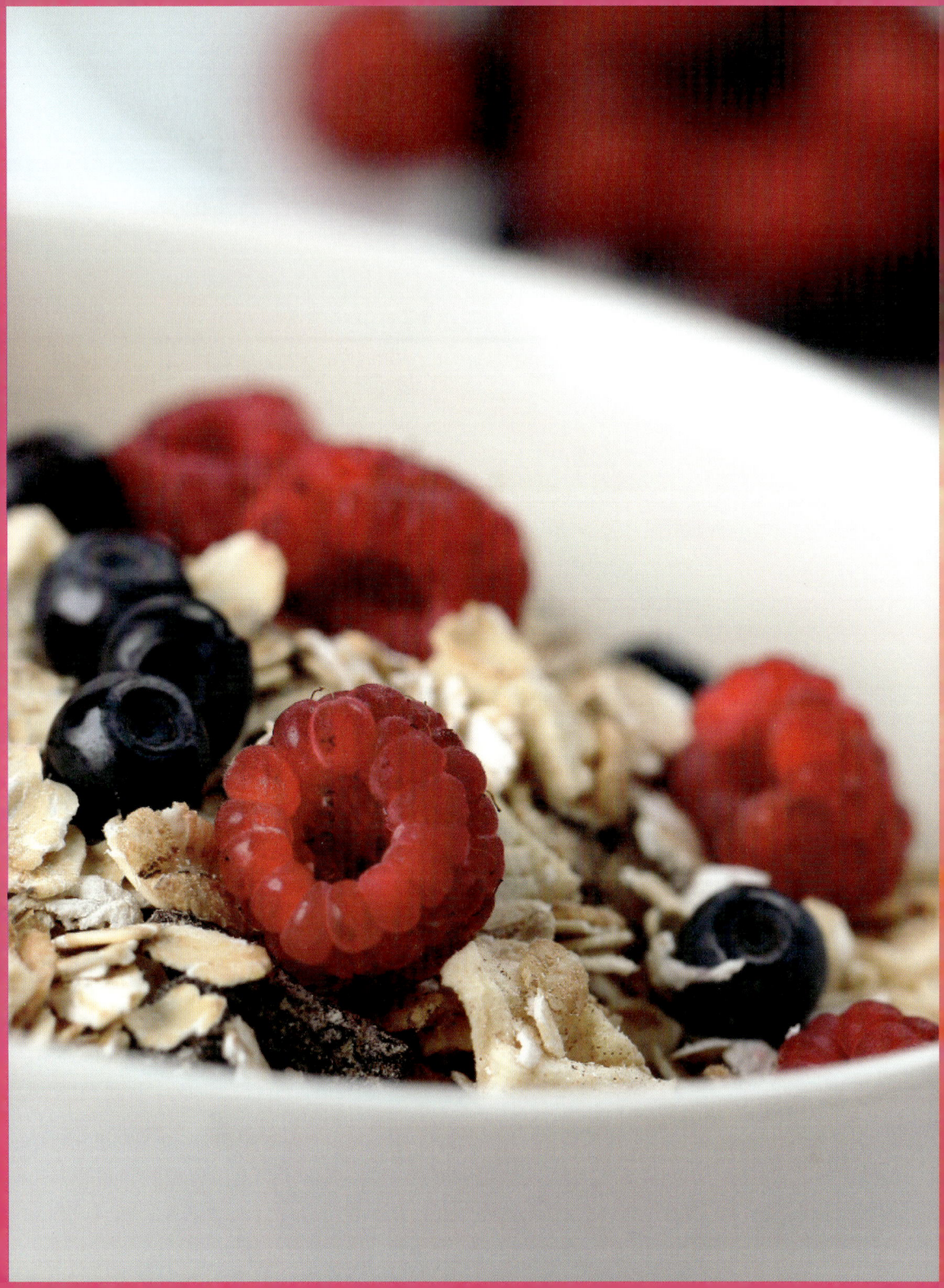

Simply Sinless Oats & Fruit

INGREDIENTS

1/3   cup uncooked oatmeal (the less processed the better)
1/3   cup nonfat plain Greek yogurt or low-fat cottage cheese
½   teaspoon vanilla extract
¼   cup blueberries, fresh or previously frozen
¼   cup raspberries, fresh or previously frozen
1   packet Truvia
1   tablespoon granola cereal (I prefer Nature's Path with flax and pumpkin)
       Drizzle of honey

DIRECTIONS

1. Combine uncooked oats, yogurt, vanilla, blueberries and Truvia in a bowl and mix until well coated.

2. Top with the tablespoon of granola cereal and drizzle with honey. Serve and enjoy!

   Serves 1.

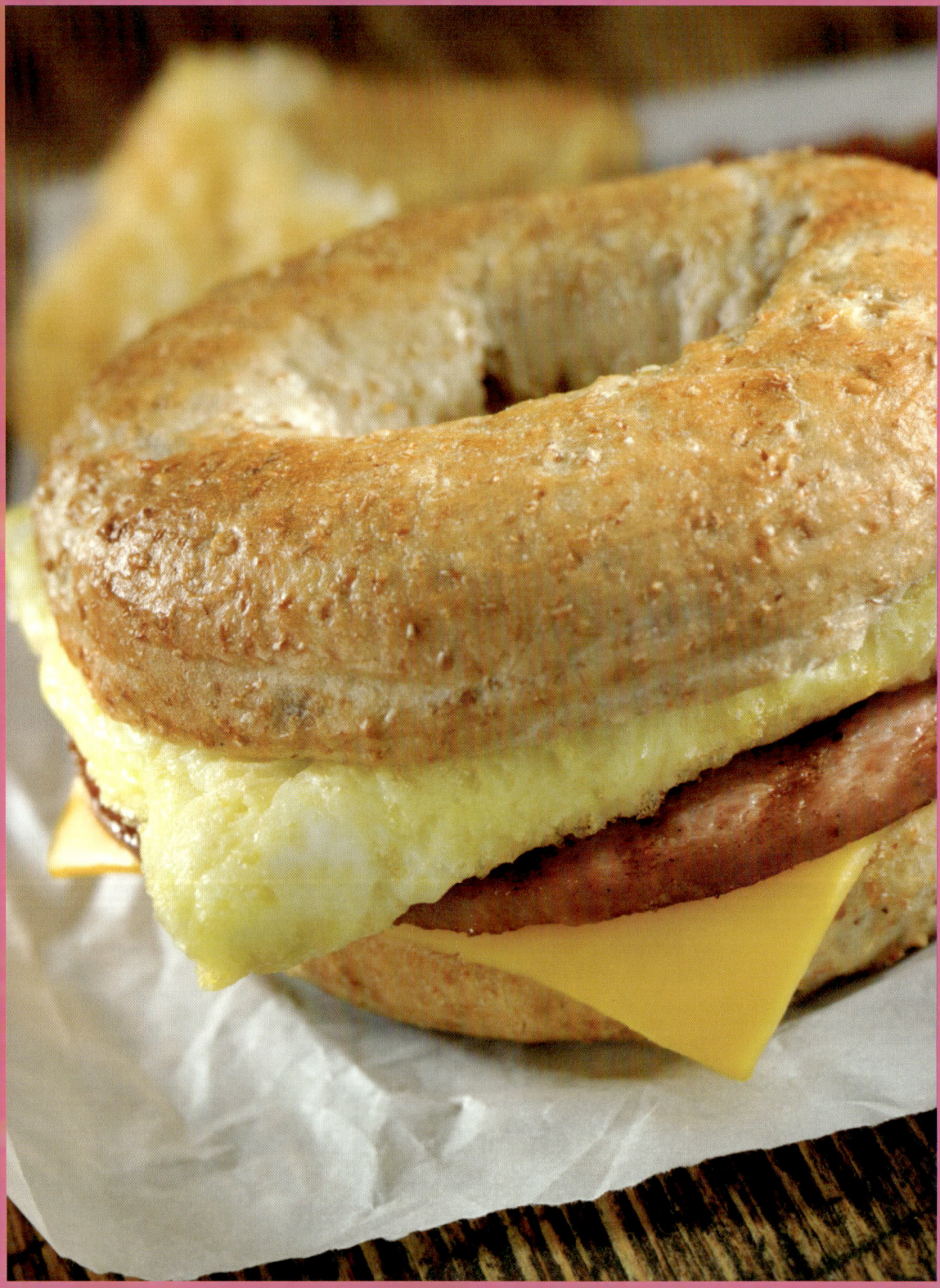

Eggs Over My Hammy Breakfast Sandwich

INGREDIENTS

1 Thomas Everything Bagel Thin

2 egg whites

3 pieces of thinly sliced deli ham or chicken

¼ cup chopped green onion

1 tablespoon low-fat cream cheese

½ piece reduced-fat cheddar cheese

Salt

Cracked black pepper

DIRECTIONS

1. Toast the bagel while cooking the egg whites and chopped green onions in a nonstick skillet sprayed with fat-free cooking spray.

2. Spread low-fat cream cheese on bottom half of bagel, top with cooked egg whites and green onion, and add salt and pepper to taste.

3. Microwave the ham or chicken for 30 seconds and place on bottom half of bagel, add reduced-fat cheddar, add bagel top, and serve warm.

Serves 1.

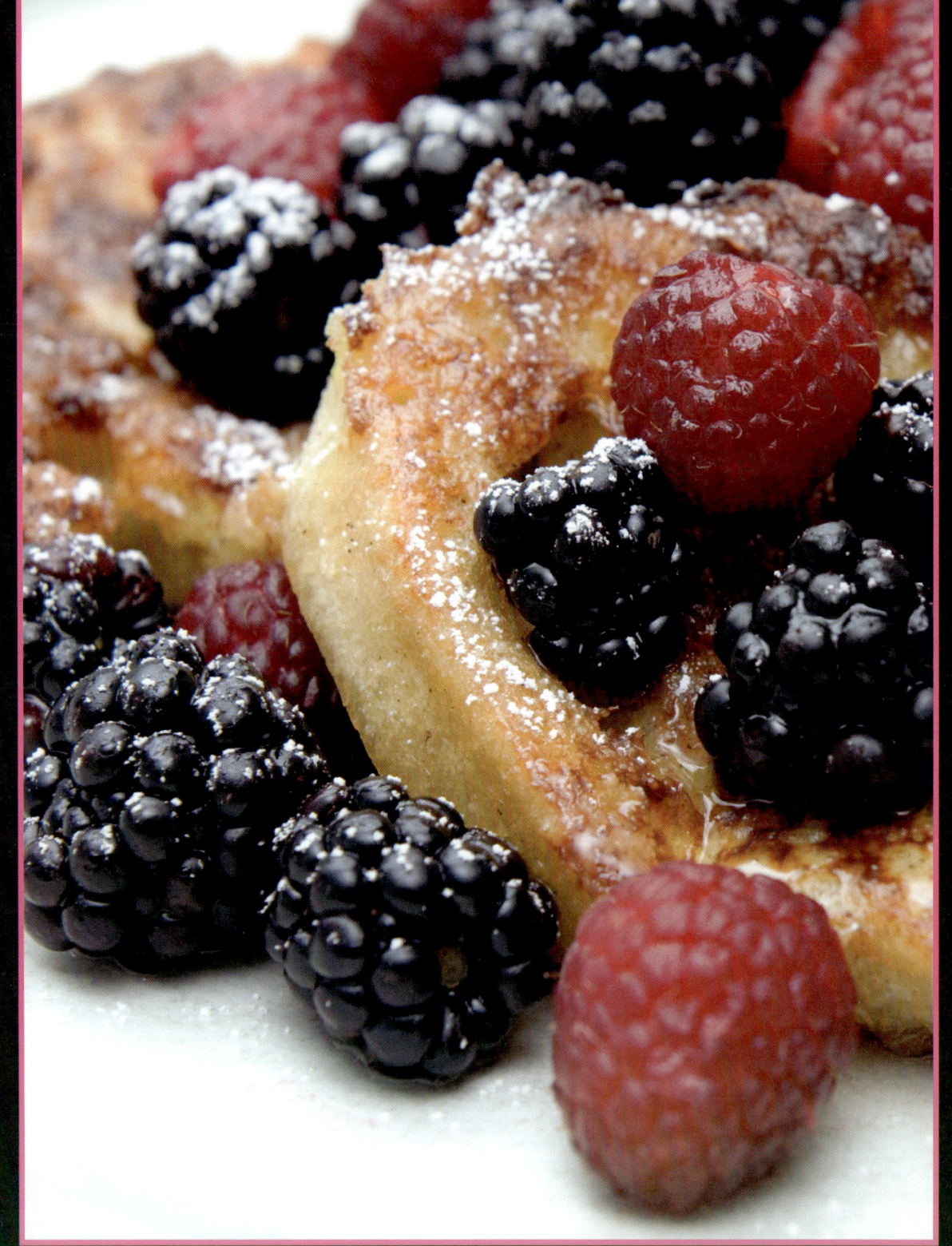

Simply Sinless Cinnamon Raisin French Toast

INGREDIENTS

4   slices Pepperidge Farm 90-calorie Cinnamon Raisin Bread
5   large egg whites
1/2 cup 1% or skim milk
1   teaspoon vanilla extract
½   teaspoon cinnamon
2   packets Truvia
      Fresh berries if desired
      Nonstick fat-free cooking spray

DIRECTIONS

1. Whisk together the egg whites, milk, vanilla, cinnamon and 1 packet of Truvia in a bowl until thoroughly mixed.

2. Preheat a nonstick skillet on medium high heat.

3. Quickly dip each slice of bread in egg mixture, making sure to coat both sides.

4. Spray pan lightly with nonstick spray and place each slice of bread onto pan, flipping once to ensure that both sides are cooked until golden.

5. Transfer to a plate, add fresh berries, sprinkle with remaining packet of Truvia, and enjoy!

Serves 2.

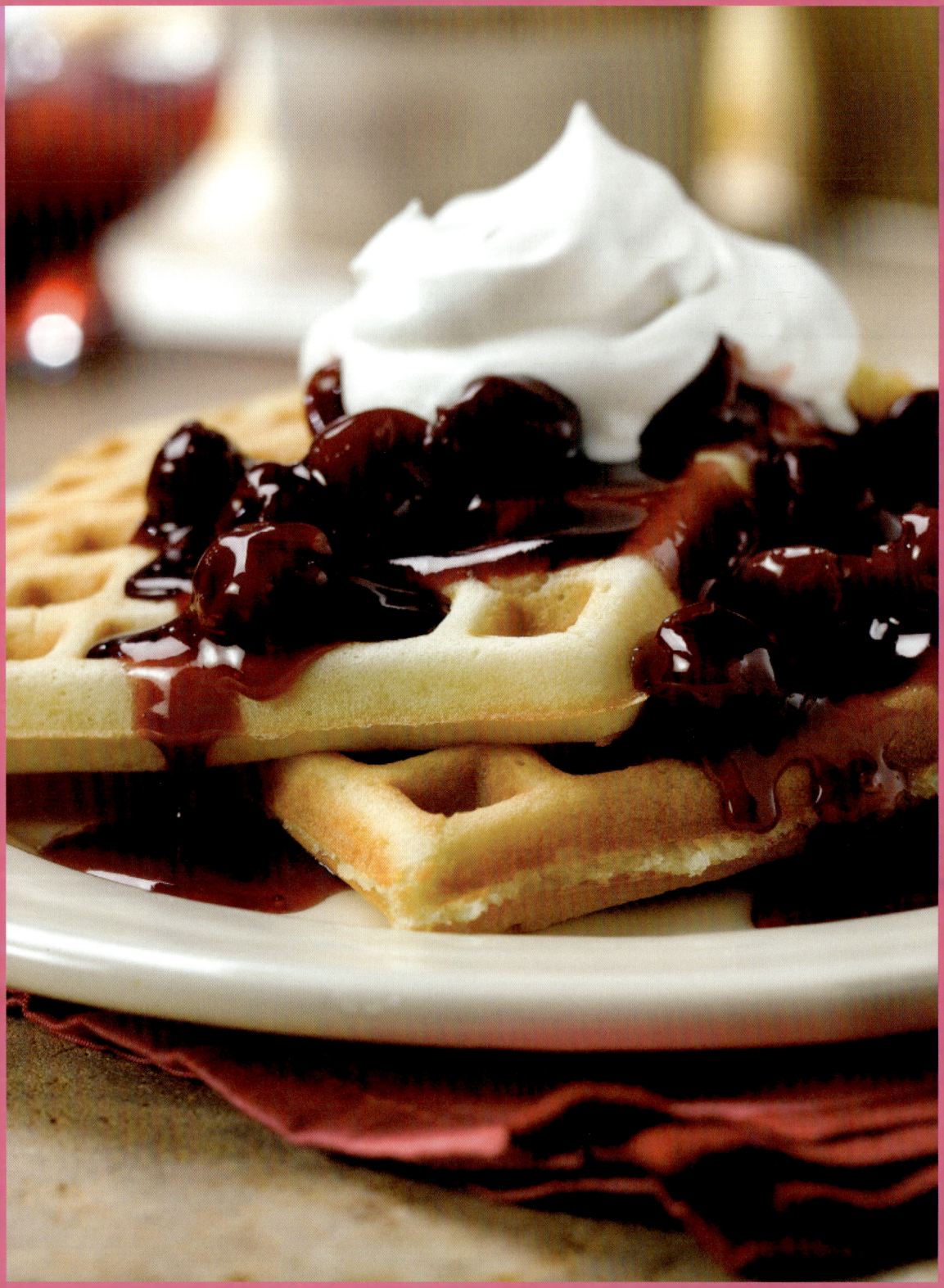

Simply Sinless *(and Super Quick!)* Berries & Maple Waffles

INGREDIENTS

2   frozen NutriGrain whole grain low-fat waffles

½   cup low-fat or fat-free Greek yogurt

1   cup fresh mixed or previously frozen berries

1   packet Truvia

1   tablespoon reduced sugar maple syrup

DIRECTIONS

1. Toast waffles.

2. Top with yogurt and berries and sprinkle with Truvia.

3. Drizzle with reduced sugar maple syrup and serve immediately.

Serves 2.

Simply Sinless Ham & Cheese Omelet with Fruit

INGREDIENTS

3 egg whites
½ cup grated reduced-fat
        cheddar cheese
4 slices of lean deli ham
        Salt
        Black cracked pepper
        Fat-free cooking spray

1 cup mixed berries
1 packet Truvia
½ *Thomas* Whole Wheat
        English Muffin
        I Can't Believe It's Not Butter
        cooking spray
2 teaspoons "All Fruit" jam
        (I prefer Polaner)

DIRECTIONS

1. Microwave ham for 30 seconds and set aside. Cook egg whites in a nonstick skillet coated with cooking spray until they set. Add cheese and ham along center of omelet, add salt and pepper to taste, and fold over. Slide onto plate and let melt.

2. Mix berries and Truvia in a small bowl until well coated, then place alongside the omelet.

3. Toast Thomas Whole Wheat English Muffin, spray lightly with cooking spray, and spread with jam. Serve immediately!

Serves 1.

Southern Bacon & Cheese Hash

INGREDIENTS

6 bacon slices

1 cup chopped white onion

2 garlic cloves, minced

1 32-ounce package frozen Southern-style hash brown potatoes

1 cup pre-shredded reduced-fat cheese blend, divided

3/4 cup chopped green onions

1/2 cup fat-free sour cream

1/2 teaspoon salt

1/2 teaspoon freshly ground black pepper

1 10.75-ounce can reduced-sodium, low-fat, or fat-free cream of mushroom soup (do NOT add water)

Fat-free cooking spray

DIRECTIONS

1. Cook bacon in a large nonstick skillet over medium heat until crisp. Pour out drippings, remove bacon from pan, and crumble. Add 1 cup onion and garlic to pan and cook for 4-5 minutes or until tender, stirring frequently. Stir in the potatoes, cover, and cook on low to medium heat for 15 minutes, stirring occasionally.

2. Combine crumbled bacon, 1/2 the cheese, green onions, sour cream, salt and pepper, and soup in a large bowl. Add potato mixture; toss gently to combine. Spoon mixture into an 11 x 7-inch baking dish coated with cooking spray. Sprinkle with remaining 1/2 cup of cheese. Cover with foil coated with cooking spray.

3. Preheat oven to 350 degrees.

4. Bake casserole, covered, at 350 degrees for 30 minutes. Uncover and bake an additional 30 minutes or until bubbly around edges or cheese begins to brown.

Serves 6-8.

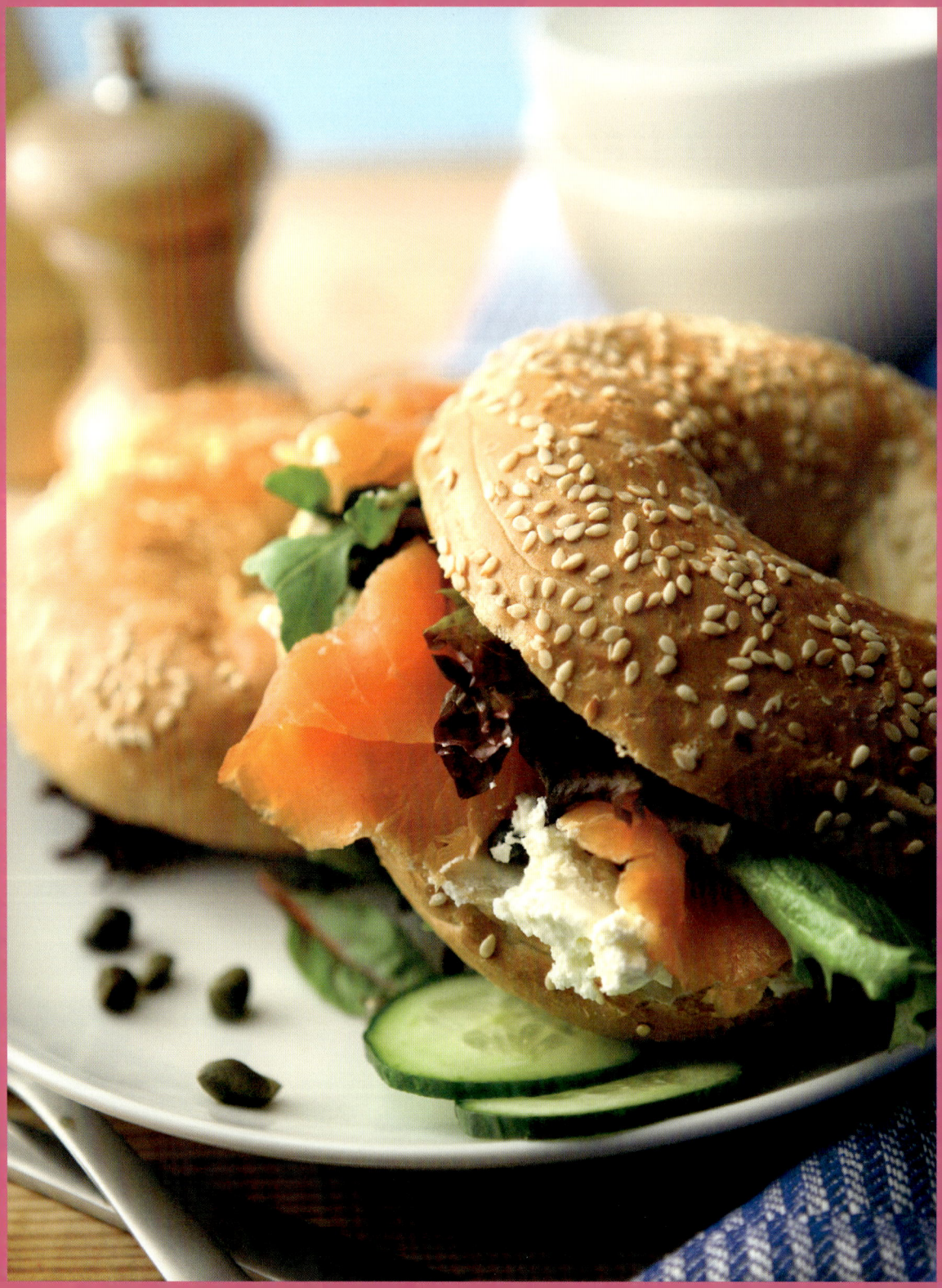

Simply Sinless Salmon Bagel & Fruit

INGREDIENTS

1 Thomas "Everything" Bagel Thin

½ cup mixed greens

2 tablespoons light cream cheese

3 ounces smoked salmon

Capers

Red onion, sliced

Cantaloupe

DIRECTIONS

1. Toast the bagel and let cool.

2. Top with low-fat cream cheese, smoked salmon, capers and mixed greens and sliced onion to taste.

3. Cut two generous pieces of cantaloupe and serve alongside the bagel.

Serves 1.

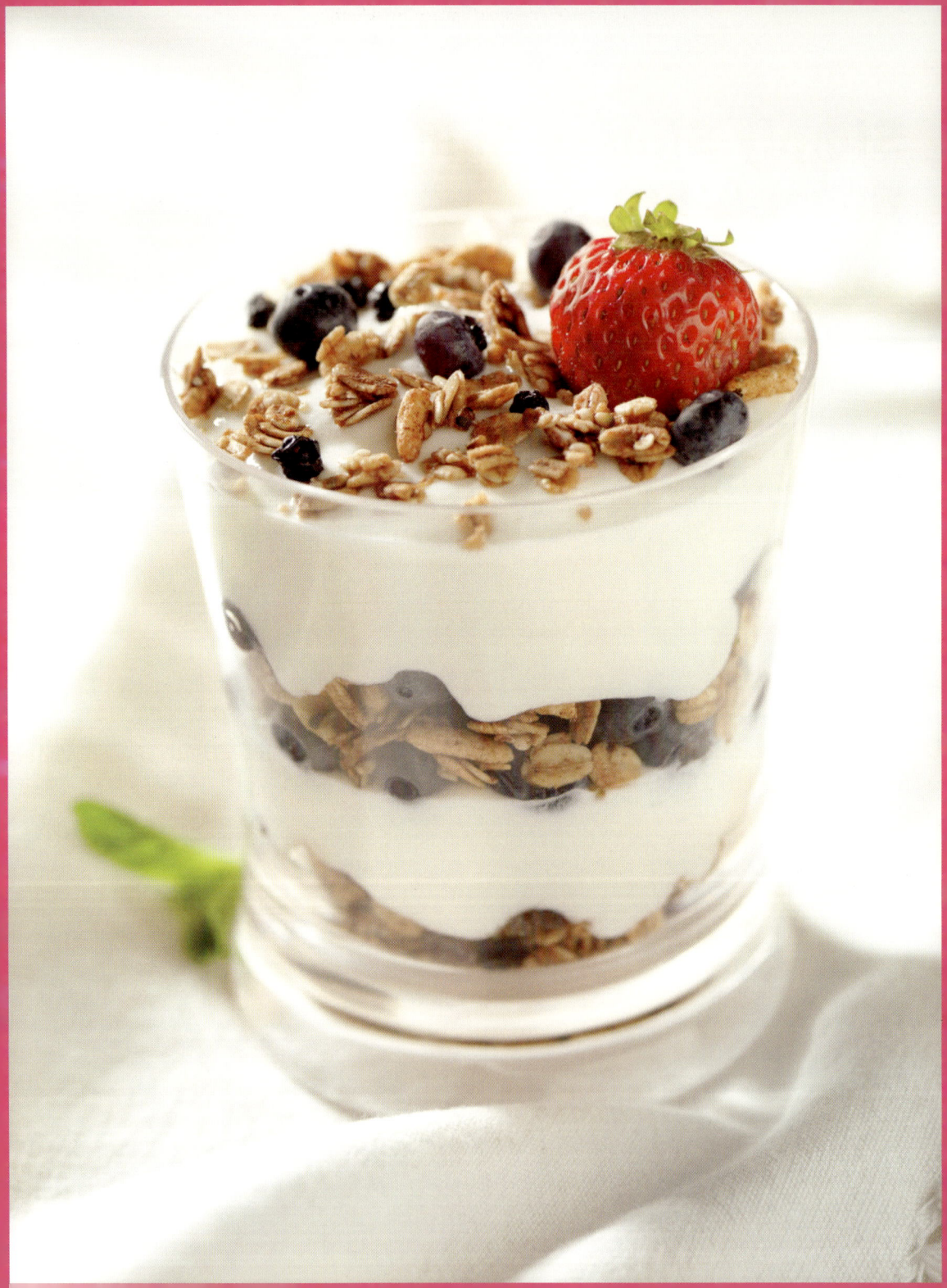

Simply Sinless *(and Superfast!)* Yogurt & Berry Parfait

INGREDIENTS

2 cups mixed berries, fresh or
    previously frozen

1 packet Truvia

6 ounces nonfat or low-fat
    plain Greek yogurt

¼ cup granola
    Drizzle of honey

DIRECTIONS

1. Mix berries and Truvia in a small bowl until well coated.

2. In a tall parfait glass or goblet, layer berries and a scoop of Greek yogurt and follow with granola. Repeat until all ingredients are used. (The top layer should be granola.)

3. Drizzle with honey and serve.

   Serves 2.

Southern Grits & Shrimp

INGREDIENTS

3 tablespoons fresh lemon juice

1/2 teaspoon Tabasco

1 1/2 pounds peeled and deveined
large shrimp

3 bacon slices, chopped

1 cup chopped white onion

1/4 cup chopped green bell pepper

1 1/2 teaspoons minced garlic

1 cup fat-free, reduced-sodium
chicken broth

1/2 cup chopped green onions, divided

5 cups water

1 1/2 cups uncooked quick-cooking grits

1 1/2 tablespoons I Can't Believe
It's Not Butter Light

1 teaspoon salt

1 cup shredded reduced-fat
cheddar cheese

DIRECTIONS

1. Combine first 3 ingredients and set aside.

2. Cook bacon in a large nonstick skillet over medium heat until crispy. Add onion, bell pepper, and garlic to drippings and cook for 5 minutes or until tender, stirring occasionally. Stir in shrimp mixture, broth, and 1/4 cup of the green onions and cook 5 minutes or until shrimp are cooked, stirring frequently.

3. Bring water to a boil in a medium saucepan; gradually add grits, stirring constantly. Reduce heat to low and simmer, covered, for about 5 minutes or until thick, stirring occasionally. Stir in butter and salt.

4. Serve shrimp mixture over grits; sprinkle with cheese and remaining green onions.

Serves 4-6.

Floor Me Florentine Breakfast Scramble

INGREDIENTS

1½ cups egg whites

½ cup freshly chopped basil

2 tablespoons reduced-fat grated Parmesan

1/3 cup chopped spinach

¾ cup petite diced tomatoes with sweet onion and garlic, drained (I like S&W)

½ teaspoon minced garlic

Salt

Freshly cracked black pepper

Fat-free cooking spray

DIRECTIONS

1. In a small bowl, stir together egg whites, basil, and reduced-fat Parmesan and set aside.

2. In a microwave-safe bowl, mix chopped spinach, tomato mixture, and ½ teaspoon of garlic; heat in microwave for about 1 minute.

3. Spray a large nonstick skillet with fat-free cooking spray, heat over medium heat, add egg mixture, and begin to scramble.

4. When eggs are close to cooked, add spinach and tomato mixture and stir until nicely mixed. Remove from heat and serve immediately.

Serves 2.

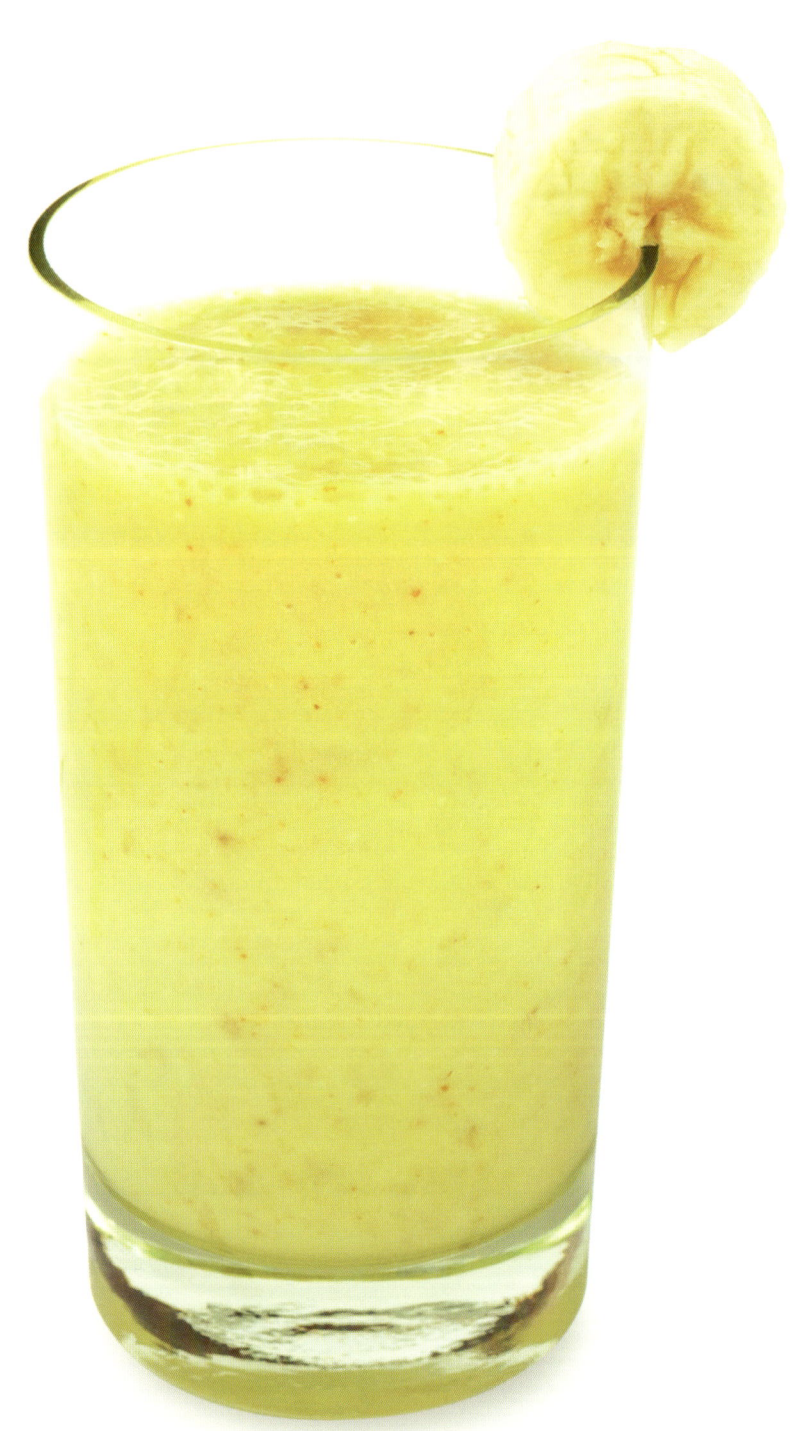

Simply Sinless Breakfast Banana Milkshake

INGREDIENTS

3 small frozen bananas (peels off and then frozen)
1 can evaporated fat-free milk
1 scoop vanilla whey protein powder
½ cup ice

DIRECTIONS

1. Peel and freeze three small to medium bananas.

2. Place three frozen bananas in a blender, add fat-free evaporated milk, and blend until smooth.

3. Slowly add 1 scoop of vanilla whey protein powder and ice, blending until creamy. Serve cold.

   Recipe is also delicious with strawberries or kiwis!

Serves 3.

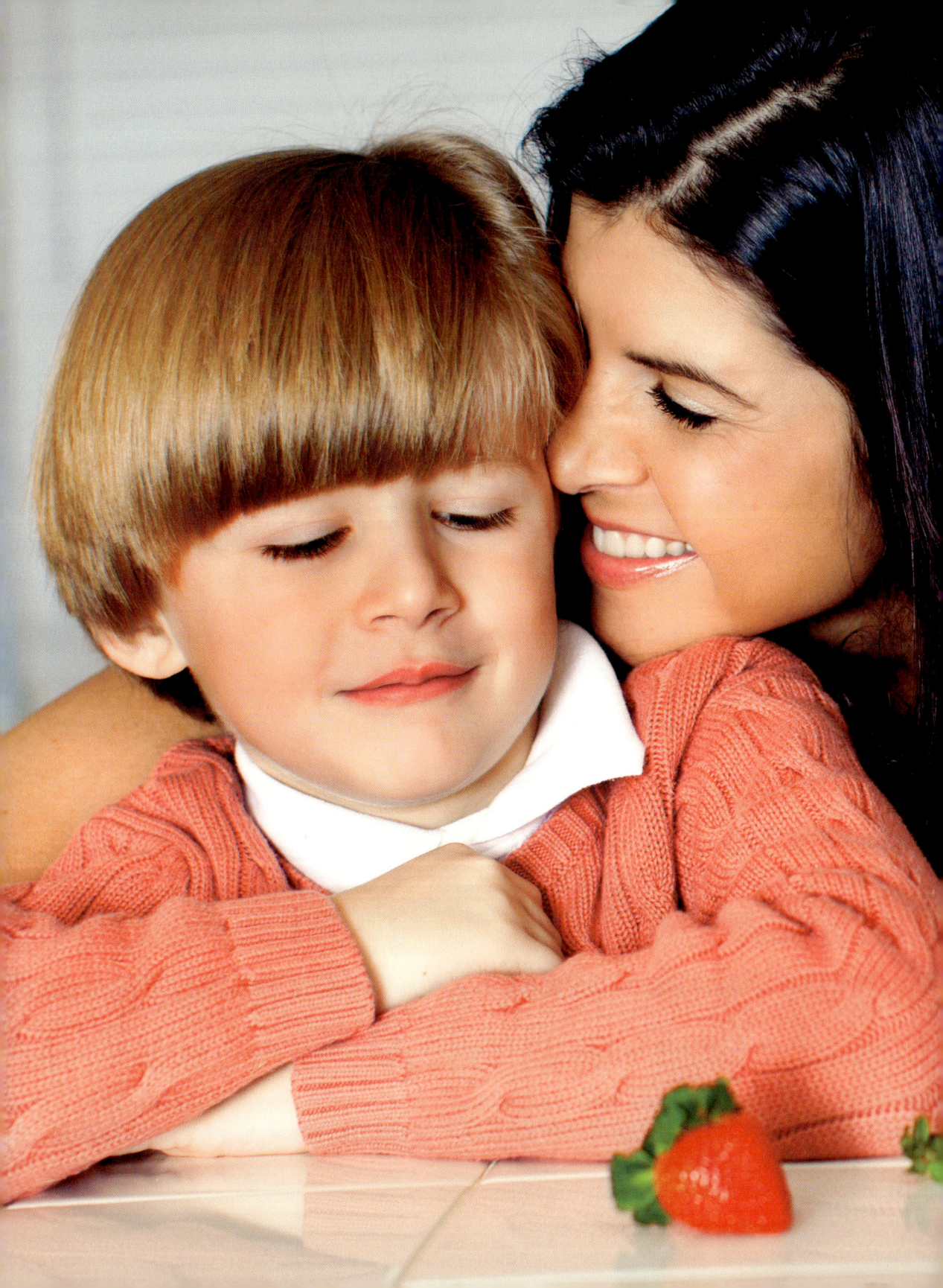

Chapter 8:

Simply Sinless Lunches

Lunch can be depressing. Who likes sandwiches day after day? These are easy, healthy alternatives to the typical mystery meat between bread slices, slathered in mayo, that we find ourselves eating day in and out.

The recipes that say Simply Sinless not only revive lunch, they make your busy life easier. With fewer than ten ingredients and requiring fewer than three steps to make, you'll be fed in no time!

Simply Sinless Teriyaki Chicken & Lettuce Wraps

INGREDIENTS

1 pound ground white meat chicken

1 10-12-ounce bag shredded carrots

5 scallions, thinly sliced

1/3 cup light teriyaki sauce (I prefer Kikkoman)

1 head iceberg lettuce

DIRECTIONS

1. Separate lettuce leaves and set aside. In a large skillet coated with fat-free cooking spray, add ground chicken, breaking up with a spatula, and cook until browned.

2. Stir in carrots, scallions, and 1/3 cup of water, lower heat to medium low, and cover. Cook until water is absorbed and veggies are soft, usually 3-4 minutes.

3. Stir in the teriyaki sauce and cook until heated through. Divide mixture among lettuce leaves and serve hot!

Serves 2-4.

Simply Sinless Turkey & Raisin Pita Sandwiches

INGREDIENTS

2   cups chopped turkey

1/3   cup diced celery

½   cup diced Gala apple

1/3   cup raisins

1/3   cup low-fat mayonnaise or
       mayonnaise substitute

Lettuce leaves

3   whole wheat pita pockets

Salt

Cracked black pepper

DIRECTIONS

1. Mix together the turkey, celery, apple, raisins, and low-fat mayo or mayo substitute and season with salt and cracked black pepper to taste.

2. Fill each pita pocket with blended turkey mixture and add one lettuce leaf to each. Serve and enjoy!

   Makes 3 entire pita sandwiches or 6 halves.

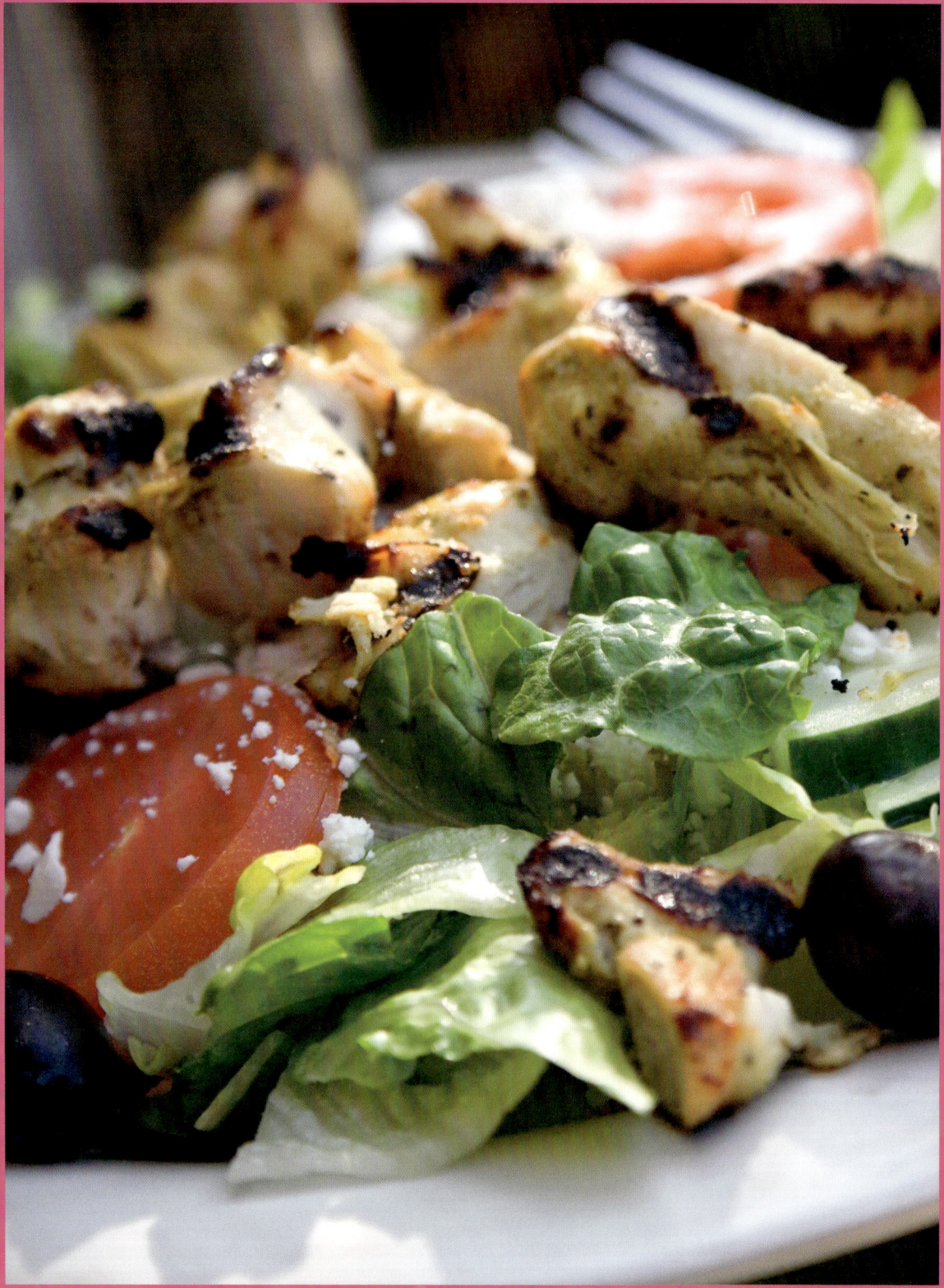

Not Good, GREAT Greek Chicken Salad

INGREDIENTS

4-6 ounces cooked chicken breast
(I take a short cut and buy it
pre-packaged)

3 cups chopped romaine

½ cup chopped green bell pepper

¼ cup chopped cucumber

5-6 halved cherry tomatoes

3 sliced radishes

1 celery stalk, chopped
Sprinkling of low fat Feta
Black or green olives for garnish
Toasted whole wheat pita or
crackers (I like Wasa crackers)

INGREDIENTS FOR DRESSING

¼ cup nonfat Greek yogurt

¼ cup reduced-fat feta, crumbled 1

½ teaspoons red wine vinegar

¼ teaspoon dried dill

DIRECTIONS

1. Prepare and combine all salad ingredients, mixing thoroughly.

2. Combine all dressing ingredients in a salad dressing shaker, toss with salad, and coat thoroughly.

3. Serve with toasted pita or crackers and garnish with 2-3 olives.

Serves 2.

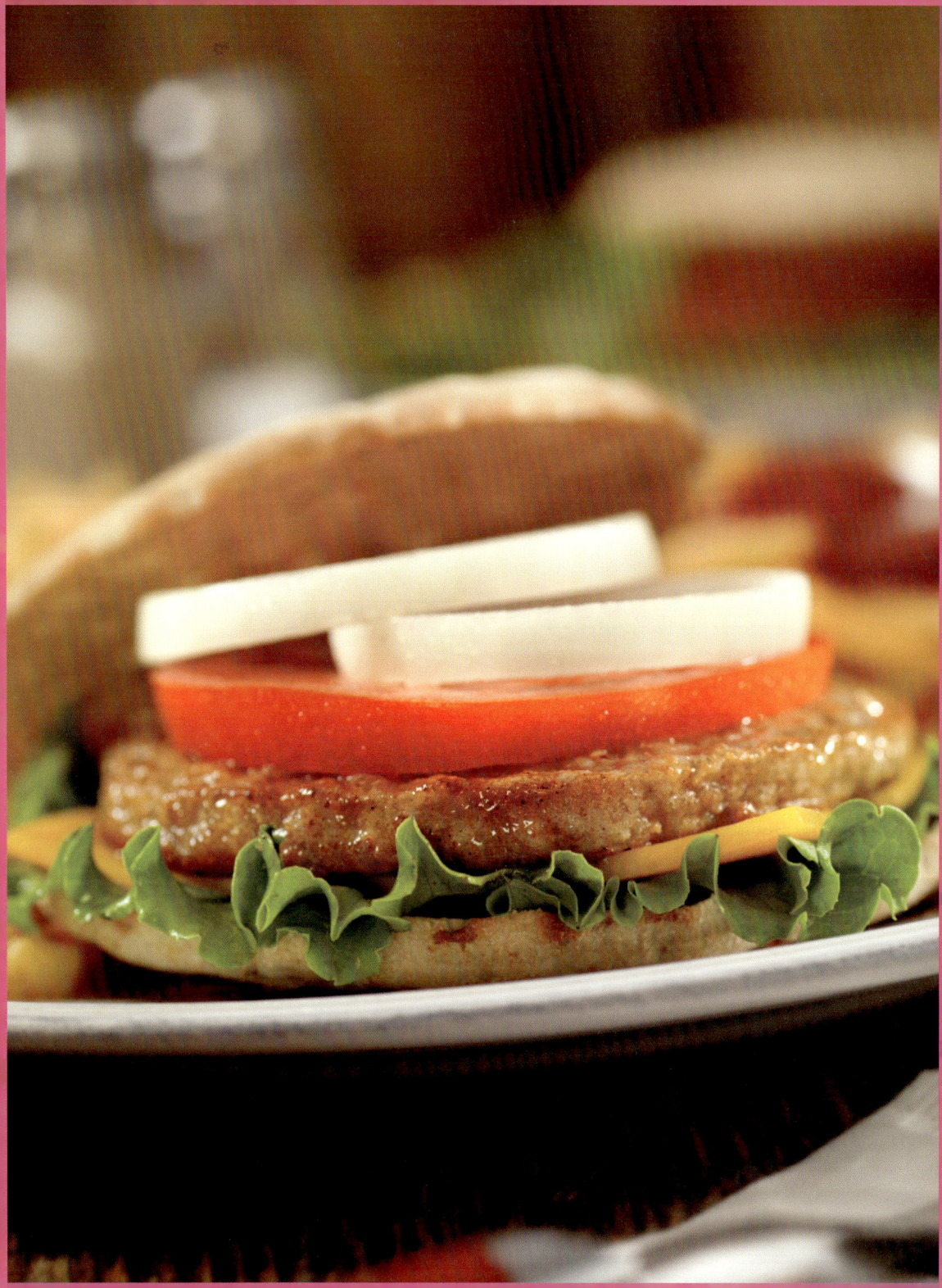

Super Fast Turkey Patty Meltdown

INGREDIENTS

1	teaspoon olive oil
1	pound ground turkey breast
¾	cup vertically sliced sweet onion such as Vidalia
¼	cup low-fat cottage cheese (or Ricotta, depending on taste preference)
2	teaspoons Worcestershire sauce
½	teaspoon cracked black pepper
1	large egg white
4	slices reduced-fat Swiss or cheddar cheese
4	slices whole wheat OR light rye bread
1/3	cup Dijon mustard, spicy country style if available

DIRECTIONS

1. Heat oil in a nonstick skillet over medium heat, add onion, and cook until lightly browned. Transfer to a plate and set aside.

2. Preheat broiler and combine turkey, cottage cheese, Worcestershire, and egg white, mixing thoroughly until well blended. Divide into four equal portions and shape patties, then return pan to medium heat and coat with nonfat cooking spray.

3. Add patties to pan and cook until brown, 3-5 minutes, then turn patties over and cook for another minute. Add 1 slice of Swiss cheese to each patty and cook until cheese begins to melt onto patty.

4. In a single layer, place bread on a broiling sheet and into broiler for 2 minutes or until toasted. Coat each piece of bread with spicy mustard and top each with a patty, then top each patty with the onion mixture and serve warm.

Serves 2.

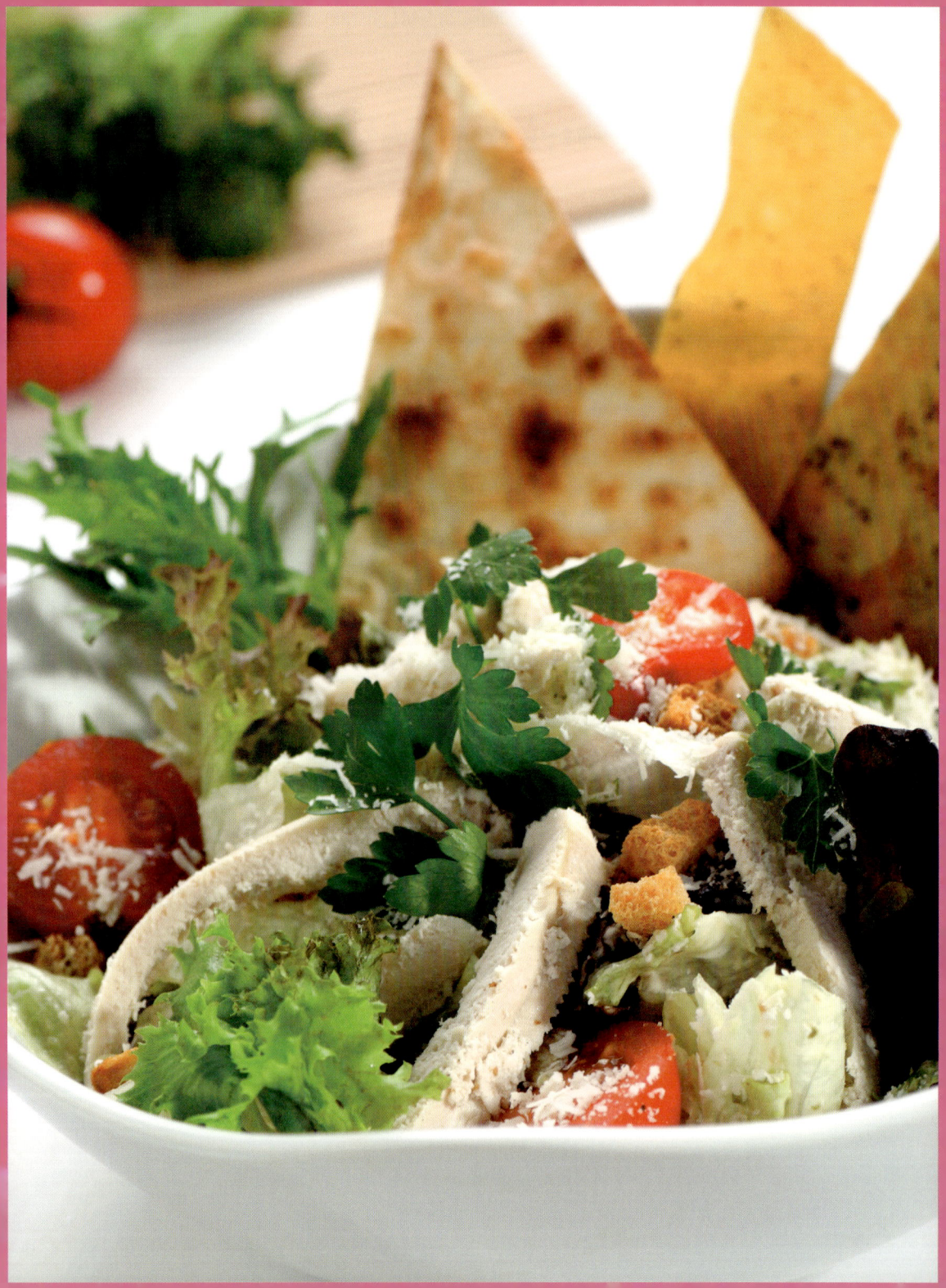

Simply Sinless Non Traditional Chicken Caesar Salad

INGREDIENTS

4 ounces grilled chicken breast (I grill extra chicken breasts on Sunday nights and use them all week in various recipes)

3 cups baby greens

½ cup whole grain fat-free croutons

4-6 cherry tomatoes, halved

3 slices red onion

1 tablespoon reduced-fat grated Parmesan

2-3 tablespoons reduced-fat or low-fat Caesar dressing

½ whole wheat pita, toasted

Flat leaf parsley for garnish

DIRECTIONS

1. Toss chopped chicken breast, romaine, croutons, tomatoes, onion, and Parmesan together until well blended. Toast the pita.

2. Drizzle salad with low-fat Caesar dressing and serve pita alongside.

Serves 1.

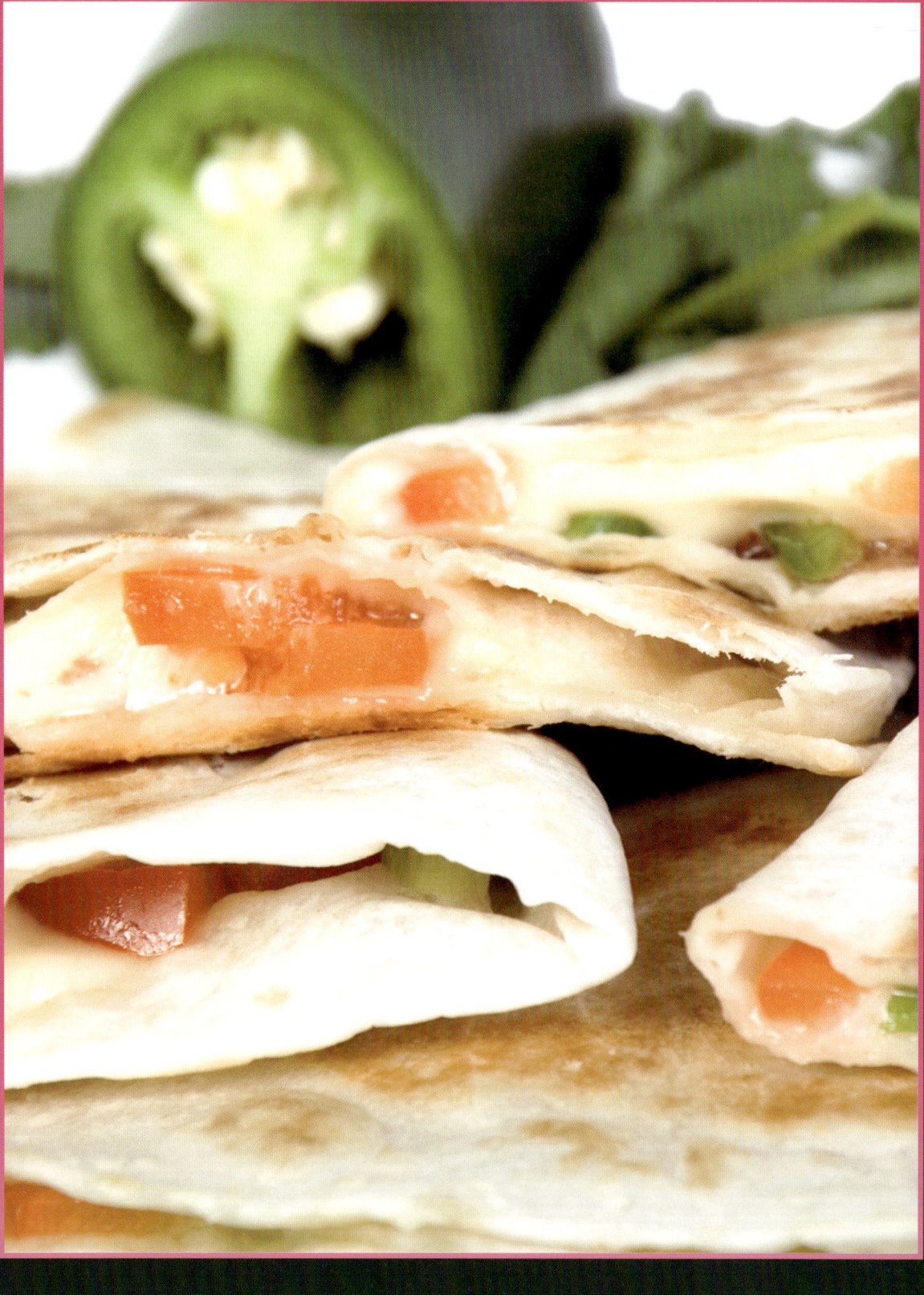

Three C's Quesa D's

(chiles, corn, and cheese...This recipe makes a nice vegetarian option!)

INGREDIENTS

2	Anaheim chiles
1 ½	teaspoons olive oil
1 ¼	cups sliced Shitake mushrooms
1	cup whole kernel previously frozen corn
½	cup chopped green onions
¼	teaspoon salt
¼	teaspoon ground black pepper

4 8-inch tortillas, preferably whole wheat

1 cup shredded reduced-fat sharp cheddar or white cheese

Fat-free cooking spray

¾ cup salsa, preferably without HFCS

DIRECTIONS

1. Preheat broiler. Cut chiles in half lengthwise, scooping out seeds and inner gook. Place chile halves, skin side up, on a baking sheet lined with foil, then flatten each chile by hand or with a wooden rolling pin. Broil 6-8 minutes until nicely browned or almost blackened. Place in a large plastic bag to allow moisture to accumulate from the heat, about 15 minutes. Remove from bag, peel, and chop, then reduce oven temperature to 225 degrees.

2. Heat oil in a nonstick pan over medium heat. Add mushrooms and sauté 2-3 minutes. Add corn, onions, salt, and pepper, and sauté another 2-3 minutes. Place corn mixture in a large bowl and add chopped chiles.

3. Take the 4 tortillas and evenly add the mushroom and cheese mixtures to 1 side of each tortilla. Place a tortilla in the skillet and cook over medium heat until cheese melts and bottom is golden. Transfer to the chile pan, now coated with non-fat cooking spray, and keep warm at 225 degrees until all 4 quesadillas are cooked.

4. Cut into wedges and serve warm with salsa.

Serves 2.

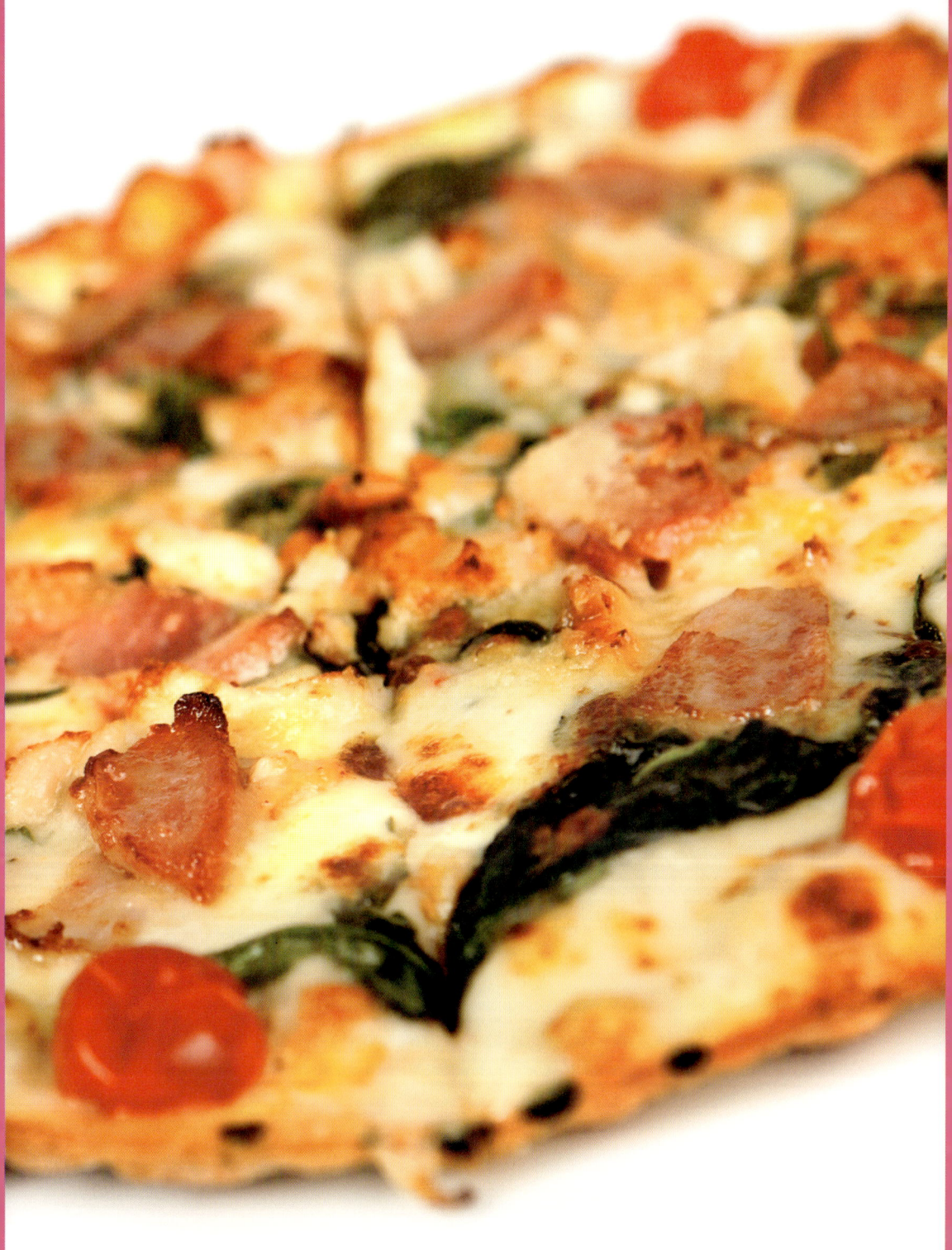

Roasted Ham and Chicken Pizza Pitas

INGREDIENTS

2   cups cherry tomatoes

2   teaspoons extra virgin olive oil

½   teaspoon Kosher salt

½   teaspoon freshly ground
         black pepper

2   12-inch whole wheat tortillas

1 ½   cups reduced-fat mozzarella
         cheese, grated

½   cup sliced lean ham

2   cups rotisserie chicken,
         skin removed

1   teaspoon dried oregano

1   teaspoon dried basil

DIRECTIONS

1. Preheat oven to 350 degrees. Toss together tomatoes, oil, salt, and pepper, then place on baking sheet and roast until blistering, usually 15 minutes. Remove tomatoes from oven and adjust oven to broil, moving oven rack to 5 inches from the broiler.

2. Place the tortillas on a baking sheet and layer each with equal portions of the cheese, chicken, and tomato mixtures. Sprinkle both with oregano and basil and broil until cheese has melted, typically 2-3 minutes. Serve warm.

Serves 2.

Superfast Chicken Pasta Salad

INGREDIENTS

8 ounces rotini (I like Barilla
Plus multigrain)

2 cups shredded rotisserie chicken
breast, skin removed

1 small red onion

2 ½ tablespoons finely chopped
fresh oregano

½ teaspoon extra virgin olive oil

1/3 cup low-sodium chicken broth

4 tablespoons white balsamic vinegar

1 can black beans, drained and rinsed

¼ cup chopped green olives (optional)
Raisins (optional)
Fat-free cooking spray

DIRECTIONS

1. Cook pasta according to directions, typically 11 minutes, and remember to salt your water. Drain and reserve ½ cup of cooked pasta water, then return pasta to pot.

2. Heat a large nonstick skillet coated with fat-free cooking spray over medium heat. Add onion, oregano, and olive oil. Cover and cook, stirring occasionally, for 2-3 minutes.

3. Add broth and vinegar to skillet and slowly stir in chicken, beans, and olives, cooking for 2-3 minutes or until thoroughly heated. Toss chicken mixture with pasta and add reserved pasta water if the mixture is too dry. Add raisins if desired.

Serves 2.

Simply Sinless Tuna, Nuts, & Grapes on Greens

INGREDIENTS

2 cups mixed spring greens

4 ounces chunk light tuna

3 tablespoons chopped pecans

1 cup red grapes, halved

4 tablespoons low-fat raspberry
    vinaigrette dressing

DIRECTIONS

1. Mix together the tuna, chopped pecans, halved grapes, and raspberry vinaigrette until well coated and blended.

2. Serve on top of mixed greens.

   Serves 1.

Simply Sinless Shrimp & Avocado Wrap

INGREDIENTS

3	cups baby greens		**1**	teaspoon extra virgin olive oil
4	ounces cooked shrimp		**½**	cup cherry tomatoes, sliced
1 ½	teaspoons honey		**1/3**	cup diced avocado
1 ½	teaspoons Dijon mustard		**1**	large whole wheat tortilla
1 ½	teaspoons lemon juice			

DIRECTIONS

1. Mix honey, Dijon mustard, lemon juice, and olive oil in a bowl.

2. Toss baby greens, shrimp, tomatoes, and avocado, then combine the two mixtures, coating thoroughly.

3. Fold mixture into a whole wheat tortilla and fold over to "wrap."

Serves 1.

Lunchtime Taco Salad Casserole*

INGREDIENTS

1	can black beans, drained and rinsed
4	cups shredded iceberg lettuce
1	medium tomato, seeded and chopped
1 ½	cups shredded low-fat sharp cheddar cheese
¼	cup sliced olives
¼	cup green onions, sliced
1	medium avocado

½	cup low-fat sour cream
1	4-ounce can chopped green chili peppers, drained
2	tablespoons 1% milk
1	clove garlic, minced
¾	teaspoon chili powder
½	cup chopped tomato
2	cups tortilla chips, crushed, preferably low-fat

DIRECTIONS

1. In a 2-quart glass salad bowl, layer black beans, lettuce, tomato, cheese, olives, and onion. In a medium bowl, stir together avocado, sour cream, chili peppers, milk, garlic, and chili powder. Spread mixture over top of salad in glass bowl and sprinkle with chopped tomato.

2. Cover with plastic wrap and chill 2-24 hours.

3. When time to serve, mix all ingredients in bowl together and serve over crushed tortilla chips.

   *It's great to make this the night before an office potluck. Everyone loves it!

Serves 4.

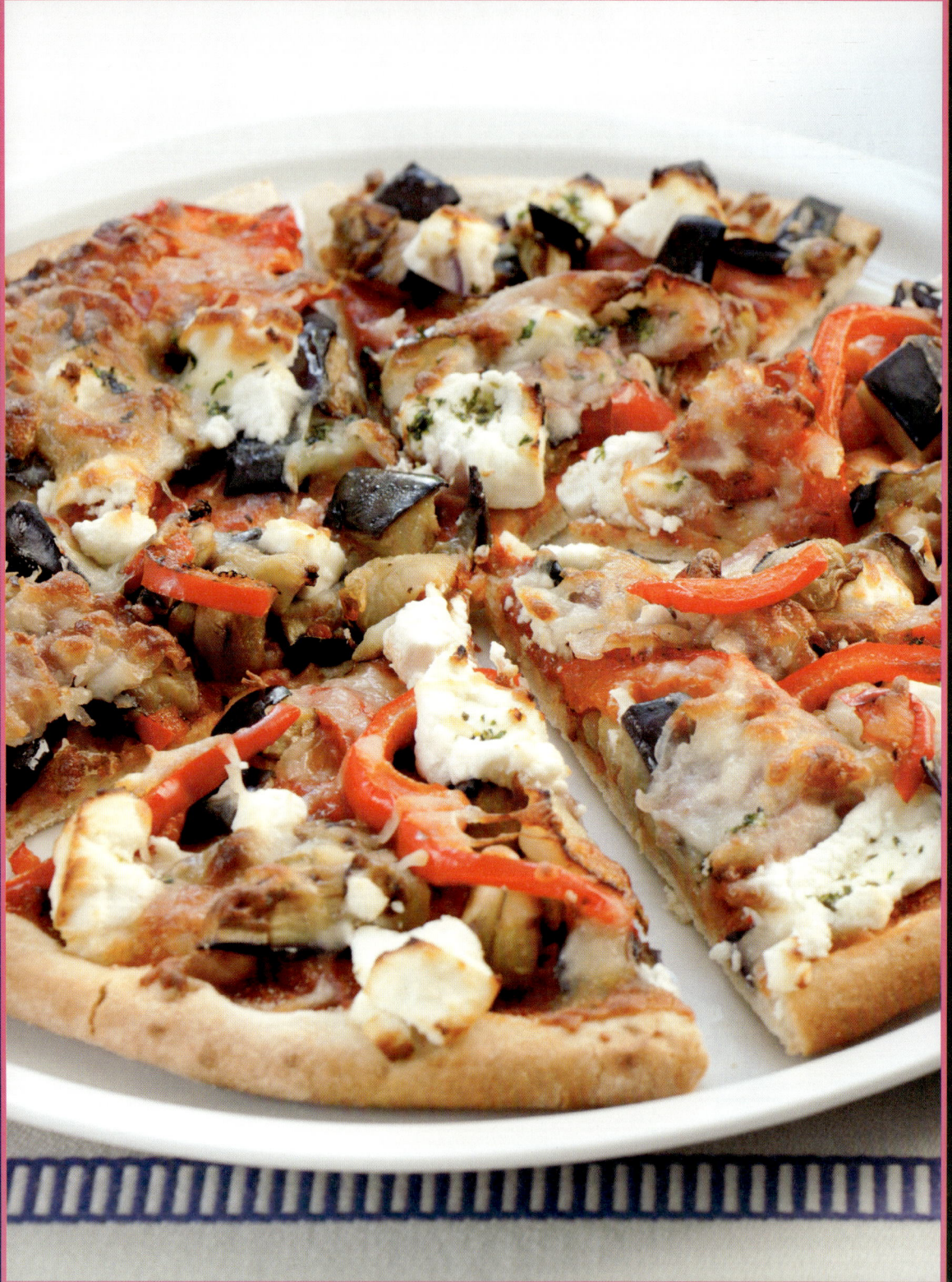

All Choked Up Chicken & Goat Cheese Pizza

INGREDIENTS

1 10-to-12-inch whole wheat
  pizza crust

4 ounces reduced-fat goat cheese

½ cup nonfat ricotta

1 cup thinly sliced chicken breast,
  rotisserie or grilled (skinless
  of course)

1 cup drained artichoke hearts,
  rinsed and halved

3 large plum tomatoes

3 tablespoons reduced-fat
  grated Parmesan

2 tablespoons fresh oregano

DIRECTIONS

1. Heat oven to 450 degrees, mix goat cheese and ricotta in a medium bowl, and spread over pizza crust, leaving about 1 to 1 ¼-inch border.

2. Top with chicken, artichokes, and tomatoes, then cover with reduced-fat Parmesan.

3. Bake until Parmesan is golden, about 8-10 minutes, top with oregano, and serve.

   Serves 2.

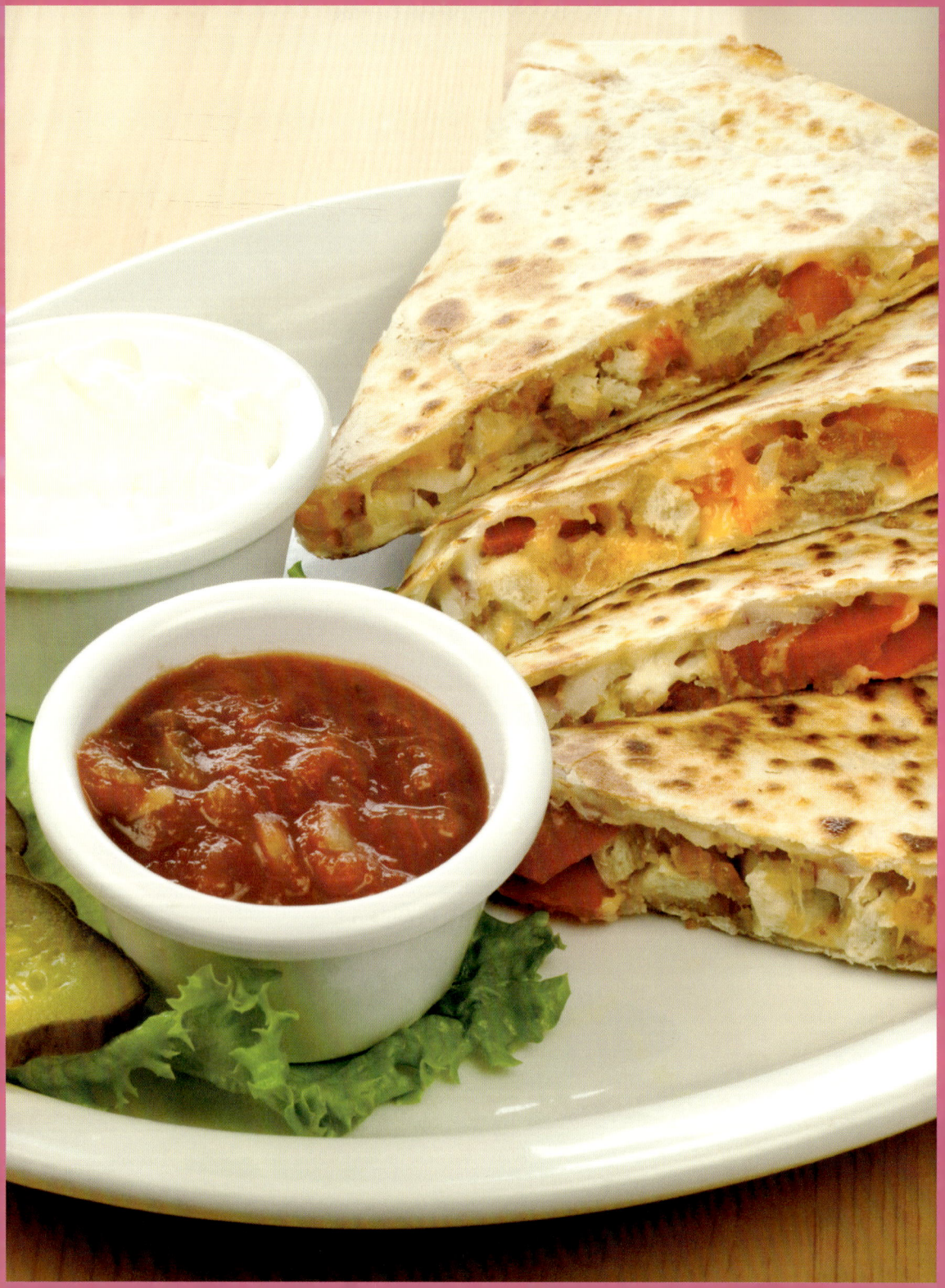

Veronica's Favorite Easy Cheesy Chicken Quesadillas

INGREDIENTS

1   cup cooked black beans

3   green onions, minced

2   garlic cloves, minced (I use minced garlic from a jar to save time)

1/2 teaspoon olive oil

4   whole wheat tortillas

2   grilled chicken breasts, sliced thinly into strips

1   large red bell pepper, roasted or grilled and sliced thinly

1/3 cup dried cranberries (my kids LOVE these in this recipe, but some people don't, so feel free to omit)

12 ounces reduced-fat cheddar cheese

1/4 cup chopped fresh flat leaf parsley

1/4 cup reduced-fat or nonfat sour cream

DIRECTIONS

1. Prepare grill and place chicken and cored red bell pepper on the top rack if available. Cook chicken 2-3 minutes per side, depending on thickness, until cooked completely. Turn the red pepper frequently to avoid scorching it.

2. Heat black beans on low (I typically heat a whole can and serve them on the side).

3. In a nonstick skillet, combine green onions, garlic, and olive oil and cook on medium until softened, roughly 3 minutes.

4. Combine 1 cup of the cooked black beans with the onion and garlic mixture and stir until well mixed.

5. Spread 1/4 of the mixed black bean mixture on 1/2 of each tortilla, followed by sliced grilled chicken, red bell pepper, cranberries, and cheese.

6. Pre-heat broiler, fold the bare half of the tortilla over the covered half, and place on a cookie sheet and into the broiler. Cook until slightly browned and crisp.

7. Cut into triangles and serve immediately while hot with the sour cream and a smidge of parsley.

Serves 2.

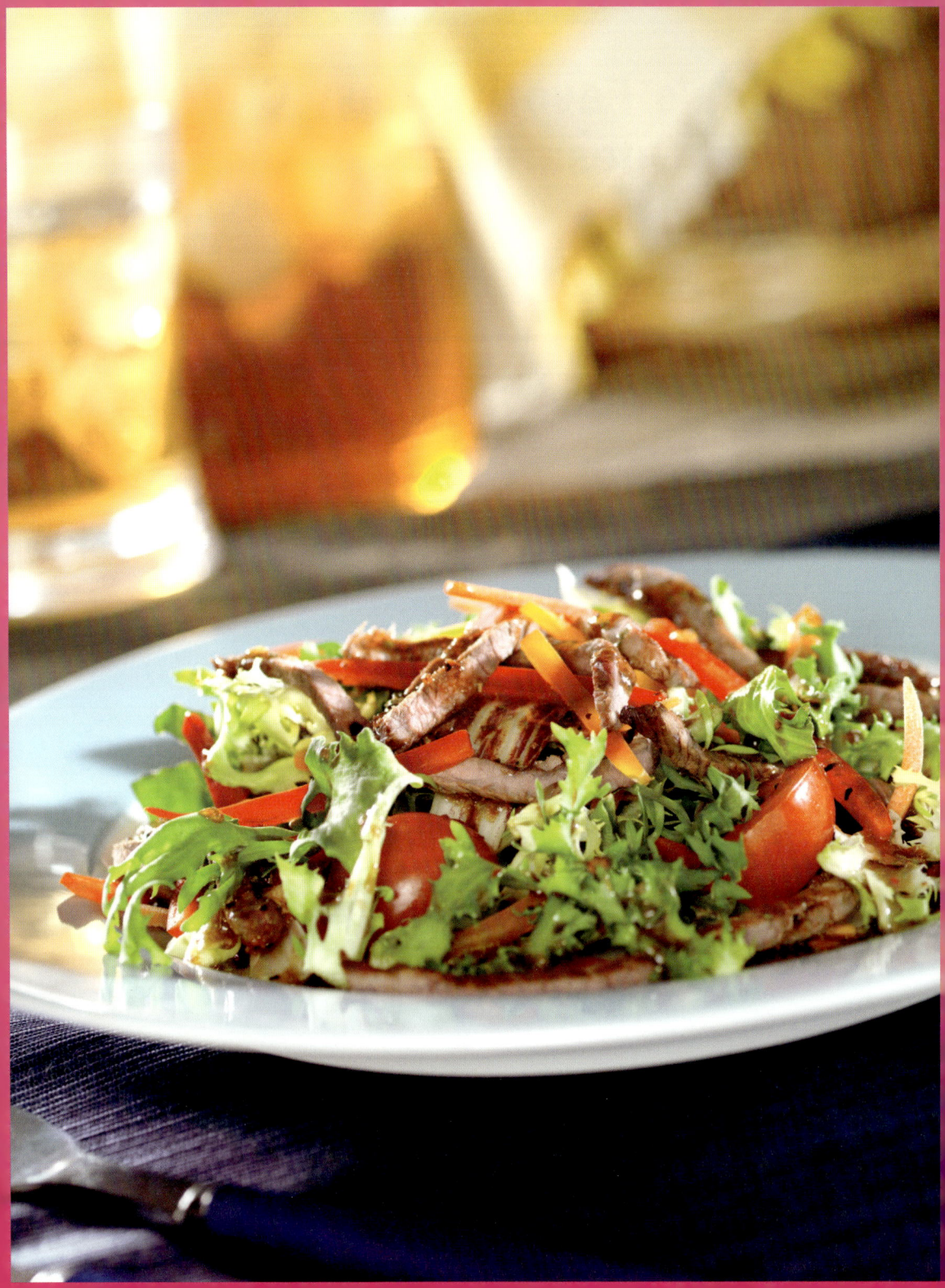

Barbequed Tenderloin Salad

INGREDIENTS

1   pound center cut beef tenderloin, trimmed and skin removed

1   teaspoon olive oil

Nonfat cooking spray

Salt to taste

Freshly cracked black pepper to taste

1   cup barbeque sauce (I use a variety that doesn't contain high-fructose corn syrup)

3-4   cups mixed greens

1 ½   cups sliced cherry tomatoes

½   cup corn (previously frozen is fine)

1 ½   cups sliced cucumber

½   cup sliced red onion

¼   cup sliced green onion

1   clove garlic, minced

1   jalapeño, chopped or sliced (leave seeds in for heat, or remove for mild flavor)

1/2   cup red wine vinegar

1   tablespoon barbeque sauce

1   teaspoon olive oil

Low-fat Ranch dressing (I love Hidden Valley)

DIRECTIONS

1. Pre-heat oven to 350 degrees. In a medium saucepan, heat 1 teaspoon olive oil and add nonfat cooking spray when pan is hot. Season tenderloin with salt and pepper to taste and sauté until all sides are seared a golden brown, about 4-5 minutes.

2. With a brush, baste barbeque sauce onto tenderloin and place in oven about 5 minutes. Repeat this process every 5 minutes for 20-22 minutes to cook the tenderloin medium rare to medium. Remove pan from oven and set aside to cool.

3. In a large bowl, mix greens, cherry tomatoes, corn, cucumber, red onion, green onion, garlic, and jalapeño. In a small bowl, mix red wine vinegar, barbeque sauce, and olive oil. Add this to the salad mixture and toss to coat.

4. Place cooled tenderloin on top of greens and serve with a side of low-fat Ranch.

Serves 2.

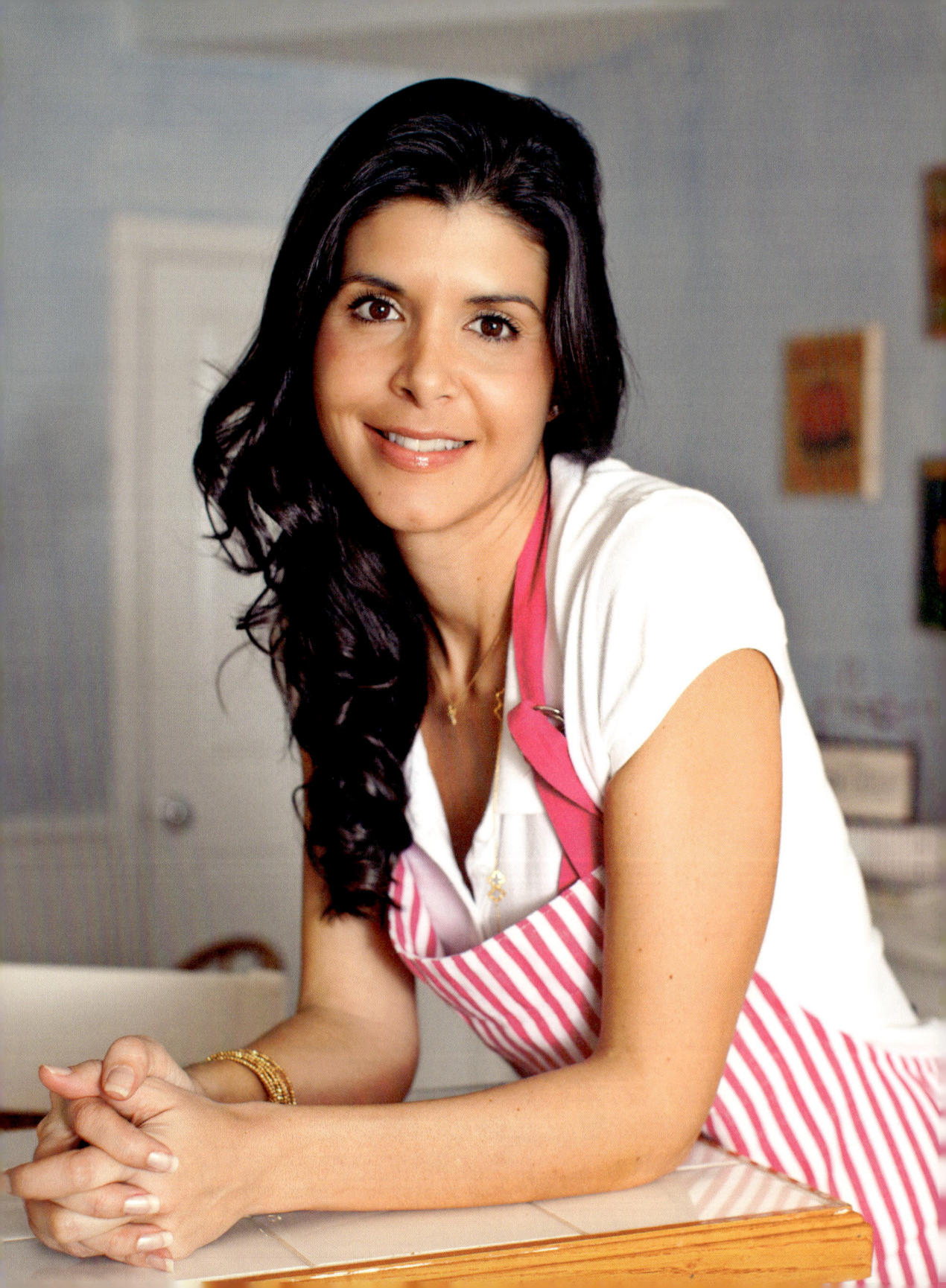

Chapter 9:

Simply Sinless Dinners

Dinnertime can be fraught with peril. After all, it's that crazy time of day when kids are doing homework and you're trying to wrap up your day while simultaneously trying to figure out what's in your fridge and what you have time to make before everyone implodes.

Stop! Before you reach for the phone to call for pizza, try out the following recipes. Specifically, head for the Simply Sinless ones on your craziest days. Remember, fast food that YOU haven't prepared = fat food. We are breaking old habits today!

There are even a few vegetarian entrees sprinkled throughout. They taste great and are a nice option for everyone, even meat lovers.

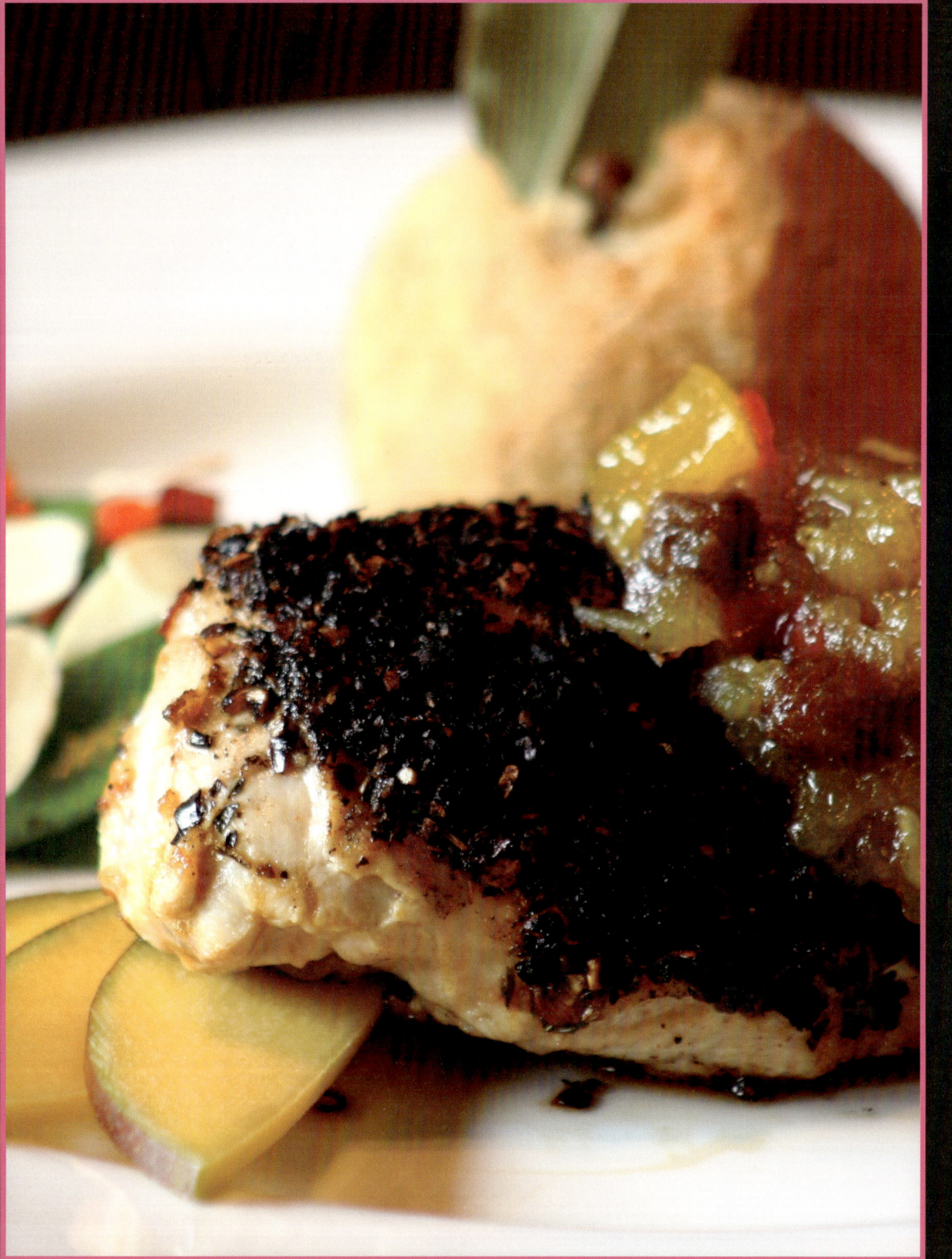

Grilled or Blackened Indian Chicken with Mango Chutney

INGREDIENTS

4	tablespoons plain low-fat yogurt
1 1/2	tablespoons paprika
1 1/2	teaspoons ground cumin
1 1/2	teaspoons ground coriander
1/2	teaspoons ground red pepper (a.k.a. cayenne)
1	clove garlic
5	teaspoons grated peeled fresh ginger
	Kosher salt

4 medium (about 2 pounds) chicken breast halves, skinless of course, pierced on both sides with a fork

2 firm-ripe mangoes

1 tablespoon light brown sugar

1 tablespoon cider vinegar

1 small green onion, thinly sliced

1 package Basmati rice, prepared as directed on box

Or fresh steamed veggies

DIRECTIONS

1. In a small bowl, mix yogurt, paprika, cumin, coriander, red pepper, garlic, 4 teaspoons ginger, and 1/2 teaspoon salt until well blended. Pour yogurt marinade into large plastic bag and add chicken, turning to coat. Seal bag, pressing out excess air. Place bag on plate and refrigerate chicken at least 1 hour or up to 4 hours.

2. Prepare outdoor grill for covered medium heat. Peel mangos and cut lengthwise; slice from each side of long flat seed as close to the seed as possible. Cut away remaining flesh from around the seed in as few pieces as possible. Place mango pieces on hot grill rack and cook about 6-8 minutes or until lightly charred and tender, turning over halfway through grilling. Transfer mangos to cutting board and set aside until cool enough to handle.

3. Chop grilled mangos and place in medium bowl. Add sugar, vinegar, green onion, 1/4 teaspoon salt, and remaining 1 teaspoon ginger; stir to combine. (Makes about 2 cups chutney.)

4. Remove chicken from marinade; discard unused marinade. Place chicken on hot grill rack. Cover grill and cook chicken 20-25 minutes, turning once until juices run clear. Slice into the thickest part of the breast if needed to ensure it's cooked through.

5. Place chicken on platter and serve with mango chutney and prepared Basmati rice.

6. Serve hot and enjoy.

Serves 4.

Orange Soy Tofu with Rice Noodles *(vegetarian friendly)*

This is healthy, vegetarian, and super yummy. Try this recipe for a break from meat.

INGREDIENTS

1 box rice noodles

1 12-ounce package firm tofu (I prefer the reduced-fat version if I can find it)

3 tablespoons rice vinegar

3 tablespoons orange juice

2 tablespoons reduced sodium soy

1 tablespoon packed dark brown sugar

1/2 teaspoon grated orange rind

1 teaspoon sesame oil

3 tablespoons thinly sliced green onions

Crushed peanuts if desired

DIRECTIONS

1. Mix honey, Dijon mustard, lemon juice, and olive oil in a bowl.

2. Toss baby greens, shrimp, tomatoes, and avocado, then combine the two mixtures, coating thoroughly.

3. Fold mixture into a whole wheat tortilla and fold over to "wrap."

Serves 2-4.

Just Peachy Chicken with Goat Cheese Salad

INGREDIENTS

4	trimmed, boneless, skinless chicken breasts
1 1/2	tablespoons extra virgin olive oil, plus 1 teaspoon more
1	large red onion (you can also use a Vidalia)

3	peaches, cut into wedges
4	cups baby green salad mix
3	tablespoons balsamic vinegar
3	ounces reduced-fat goat cheese (I also use reduced-fat blue cheese as an alternative)
½	teaspoon kosher salt
½	teaspoon freshly cracked black pepper

DIRECTIONS

1. Fire up the grill to medium high heat and brush chicken with 1 teaspoon olive oil and salt and pepper to taste. In a large bowl, mix the onion, peaches, 1 tablespoon olive oil, salt, and pepper.

2. Grill chicken and onions 4-6 minutes per side or until juices run clear and onions are tender. Grill the peaches until lightly charred, about 2 minutes per side.

3. Mix the baby greens with the onion/peach mix, balsamic vinegar, and remaining oil, top with the reduced-fat goat cheese, and serve alongside the grilled chicken. Yum!

Serves 4.

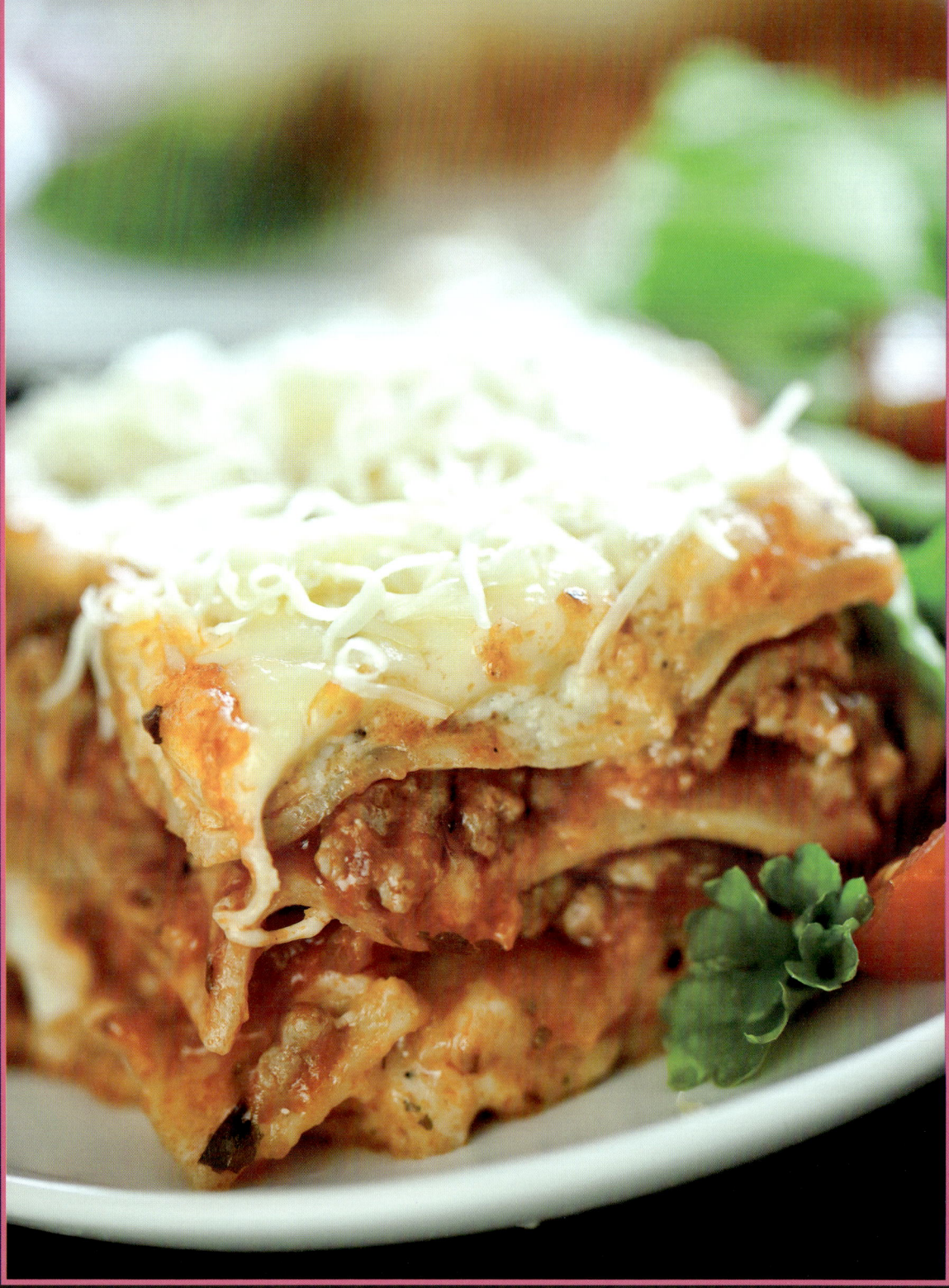

Low-Fat & Short-on-Time Lasagna

INGREDIENTS

2   pounds 93% lean ground beef
         Cooking spray
1 ½   cups water
1   jar pasta sauce (I like the Healthy Choice or Ragu Light versions)
3   cups shredded part-skim mozzarella cheese, divided
2 1/2 cups low-fat cottage cheese
3/4   cup grated Parmesan (reduced-fat if you can find it)
3/4   cup egg whites
½   cup chopped flat leaf parsley
½   teaspoon black pepper
         Oven-ready lasagna noodles (I prefer whole wheat for nutritional value)

DIRECTIONS

1. Preheat oven to 350 degrees. Cook the lean ground beef in a large saucepan coated with fat-free cooking spray over medium heat until browned. Drain off excess fat and stir to crumble. Add water and pasta sauce and bring to a near boil. Cover, reduce heat, and simmer for about 8 minutes. Remove from heat.

2. Combine 2 cups of the mozzarella, cottage cheese, Parmesan, egg whites, parsley, and black pepper in a bowl. Mix until thoroughly blended.

3. Spread 1 cup of beef mixture in the bottom of a 13 x 9-inch baking dish and arrange three or so noodles on top. Top with 1 ½ cups of beef mixture. Spread half the cheese mixture on top of beef. Continue layering noodles, beef, and cheese, finishing with one more layer of noodles and one more of beef.

4. Cover and bake at 385 degrees for 45 minutes. Then remove from oven and uncover, add remaining cup of mozzarella, and bake uncovered for 10 more minutes or until brown and bubbly.

5. Allow to cool and set for 15 minutes prior to serving.

Serves 6-8.

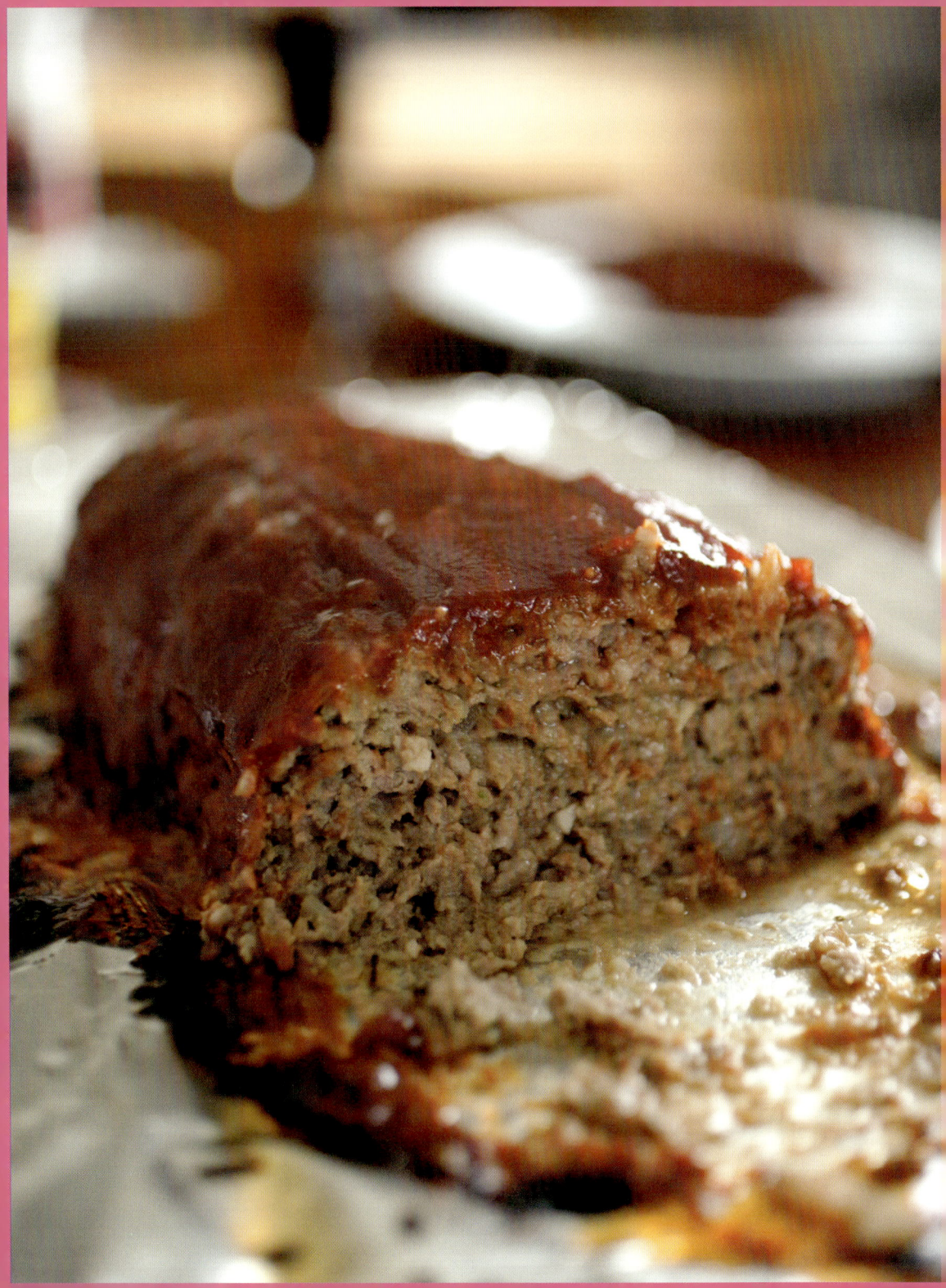

Mamaw's Meaner & Leaner Meatloaf

INGREDIENTS

2 pounds 93% lean ground beef

1 tablespoon extra-virgin olive oil

1 small yellow onion, diced

1 garlic clove, minced

1 bay leaf

1 medium red pepper, finely diced

2 tablespoons chopped fresh flat leaf parsley

2 teaspoons chopped fresh thyme

2 large egg whites, lightly beaten

¾ cup dry breadcrumbs (whole wheat if you can find it)

1 cup reduced-sugar ketchup, separated*

1 ½ tablespoons Worcestershire sauce

2 teaspoons kosher salt

1 teaspoon freshly cracked black pepper

Fat-free cooking spray

DIRECTIONS

1. Preheat the oven to 325 degrees and line a baking sheet with lightly sprayed parchment paper.

2. Heat olive oil in a skillet and add onions, garlic, and bay leaf. Sauté until tender, or about 3 minutes. Add red pepper and sauté another 5 minutes. Add parsley and thyme and sauté another 2 minutes. Remove from heat and let mixture cool, then pick out the bay leaf and toss.

3. In a large bowl, mix beef, egg whites, breadcrumbs, ½ cup reduced-sugar ketchup, Worcestershire sauce, salt, pepper, and cooled onion mixture. (You can use a spatula, but I always find that using my hands is the best way to mix these ingredients.)

4. Transfer the mixture from the bowl to the center of the parchment-lined baking sheet and form into a loaf. Spread the remaining ½ cup of ketchup across the loaf and bake for about an hour or until firm. Let cool and set for 5-8 minutes before slicing to serve. Enjoy!

Serves 8.

*Depending on the shape of your loaf, you may require more reduced-sugar ketchup for the topping.

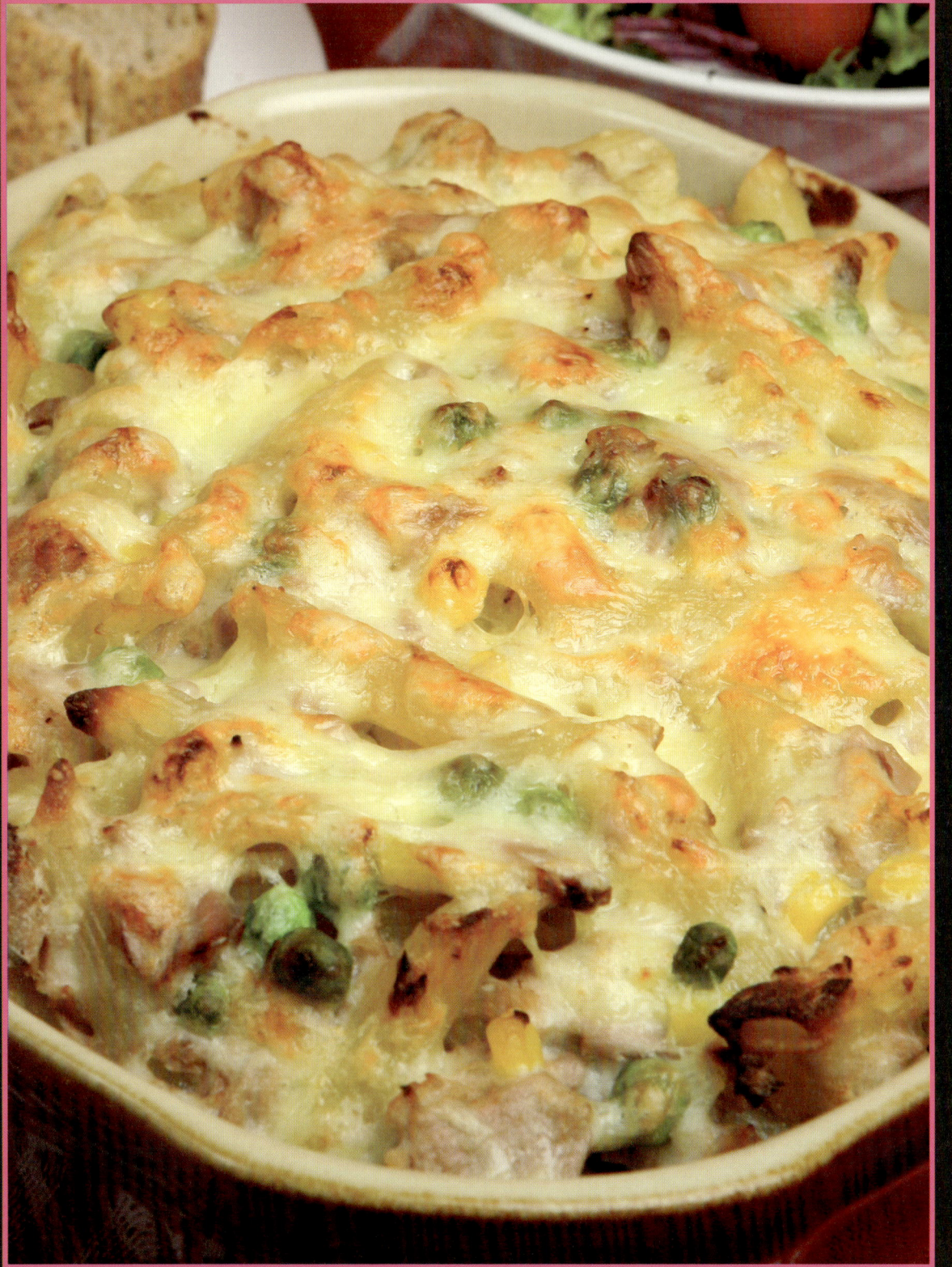

Simply Sinless & Totally Terrific Tuna Casserole*

INGREDIENTS

1 1/2 tablespoons I Can't Believe It's Not Butter Light

1 cup small onion, diced

1 cup 1% milk

1 can reduced-sodium and reduced-fat cream of mushroom soup (do not add water!)

3 cups hot cooked egg noodles

1 ½ cups previously frozen green peas

1 tablespoon lemon juice

½ teaspoon salt

½ teaspoon freshly cracked black pepper

2 cans Albacore tuna in water, drained and mixed up

2 ounces (1 small jar) diced pimiento, drained

1/3 cup whole wheat breadcrumbs

4 tablespoons reduced-fat grated Parmesan cheese

DIRECTIONS

1. Preheat oven to 450 degrees and melt butter in a saucepan over medium heat. Add onion and sauté about 3 minutes, then add mushroom soup and 1% milk. Cook for about 3 minutes, stirring constantly with a whisk so it doesn't scorch.

2. Mix soup and onion mixture with noodles, peas, lemon juice, salt, pepper, tuna, and pimiento and pour into a 2-quart casserole.

3. Mix together breadcrumbs and Parmesan and sprinkle over the top of the casserole. Bake at 450 degrees until heated through and bubbling. Serve hot and enjoy!

Serves 8.

*This is great to make on a Sunday night and refrigerate. It's perfect for those days in the week when your schedule gets away from you and you hear, "What's for dinner?"

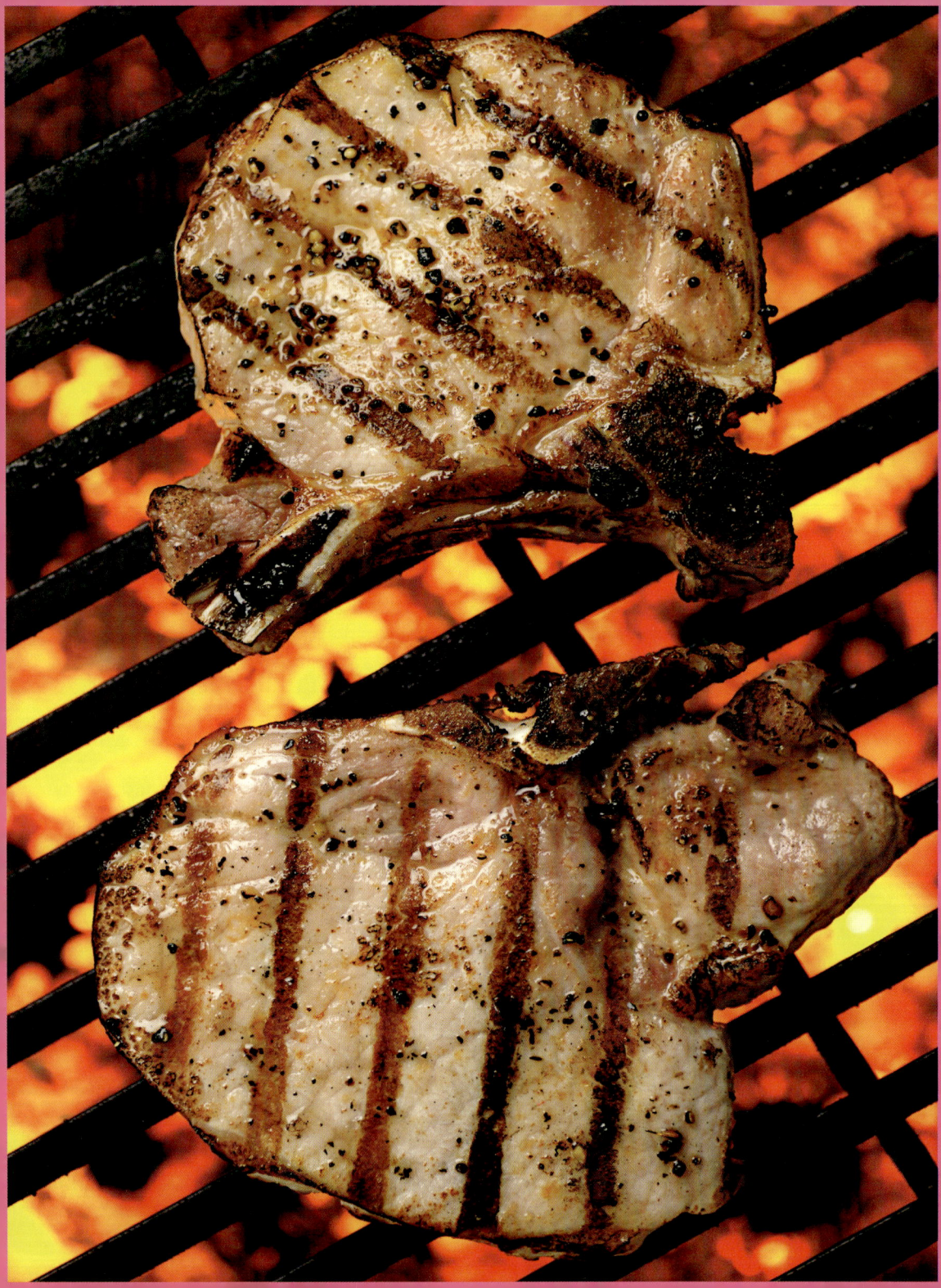

Simply Sinless Grilled Pork Chops with Maple Taters

INGREDIENTS

4 1-inch, bone-in pork chops with the fat trimmed off

2 large sweet potatoes cut into wedges

1 ½ tablespoons extra virgin olive oil

2 tablespoons reduced-calorie maple syrup (sugar-free works as well)

3 scallions, chopped

Kosher salt

Freshly cracked black pepper

DIRECTIONS

1. Fire up the grill to medium-high heat and season the trimmed pork chops with salt and pepper to taste. Grill 6-8 minutes per side or until cooked through.

2. In a large bowl, toss the sweet potatoes with the olive oil, salt, and pepper. Place on grill and turn often, watching until lightly blackened, about 10 minutes.

3. In the same bowl, add reduced sugar syrup and scallions, remaining oil, and ½ teaspoon each salt and pepper. Whisk together until well blended. Add the grilled and hot sweet potatoes and toss to coat. Brush any remaining mixture onto the grilled pork chops and serve both hot.

Serves 4.

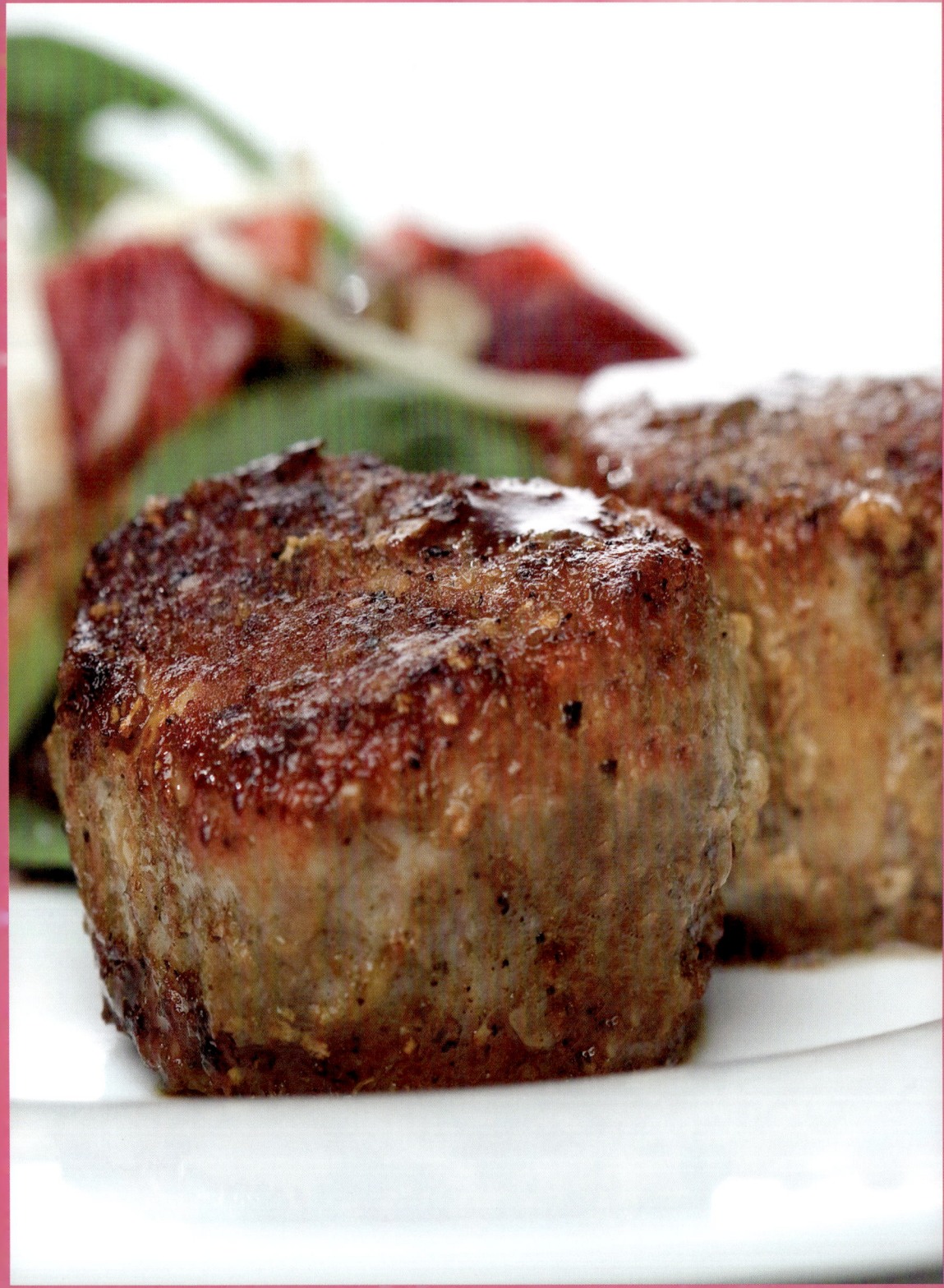

Simply Sinless Spicy Gingered Pork & Spinach Salad

INGREDIENTS

1 1-pound pork tenderloin, trimmed

1 tablespoon hot chile sauce (I like Huy Fong but other Sriracha sauces are fine)

3 tablespoons Splenda Brown Sugar Blend

1 teaspoon garlic powder

½ teaspoon salt

3 cups baby spinach or baby mixed greens

2 cups Napa cabbage, thinly sliced

1 large red bell pepper, cut into thin strips

½ cup low-fat sesame ginger dressing (I love Newman's Own) Fat-free cooking spray

DIRECTIONS

1. Preheat oven to 200 degrees. Cut pork into ½-inch slices and flatten either by hand or with a wooden rolling pin. In a bowl, mix together pork and hot chile sauce until well coated, then add Splenda, garlic powder, and salt, making sure to toss and coat very well.

2. Heat a large nonstick skillet over medium-high heat and coat with fat-free cooking spray. Add pork mixture to pan and cook until done, about 2-3 minutes per side. Remove from heat and place on a baking sheet in a warmed oven.

3. Toss greens, cabbage, bell pepper, and sesame ginger dressing in a large bowl, making sure to coat thoroughly. Remove pork from warmed oven and serve salad alongside pork.

Serves 2-4.

Simply Sinless Gingered Raisin Chicken

INGREDIENTS

½ tablespoon olive oil

4 boneless skinless chicken
   breasts (trimmed)

1 14.5-ounce can diced tomatoes

½ cup raisins

3 tablespoons lemon juice

3 tablespoons Splenda Brown
   Sugar Blend

2 ½ teaspoons freshly grated ginger (or 1
     teaspoon dried ginger)

¼ teaspoon cinnamon

½ teaspoon freshly ground
   black pepper

   Nonfat cooking spray

DIRECTIONS

1. Heat oil in a large skillet over medium-high heat, add a touch of nonfat cooking spray, and brown chicken about 3 minutes on each side. Remove from pan and set to the side.

2. In the skillet, blend tomatoes, raisins, lemon juice, Splenda, ginger, cinnamon, and pepper and bring to a boil. Reduce heat and simmer 2-4 minutes until mixture begins to thicken.

3. Add chicken breasts, cover, and simmer 12-15 minutes or until cooked through. Serve hot with a side of steamed asparagus or brown rice.

Serves 4.

Spectacular Radicchio Spaghetti (*vegetarian friendly*)

INGREDIENTS

¾ tablespoon olive oil

5 cups thinly sliced onion (I prefer Vidalia for the sweetness)

¾ teaspoon crushed red pepper

6 garlic gloves, minced

¾ cup dry white wine

1 pound uncooked whole wheat spaghetti

3 ½ cups radicchio, sliced very thinly (about 1 head of radicchio)

3 tablespoons fresh flat leaf parsley, chopped

3 teaspoons fresh oregano, chopped

1 teaspoon salt

¾ teaspoon freshly ground black pepper

1 cup reduced-fat Parmesan, grated

DIRECTIONS

1. Heat oil in a large Dutch oven over medium-high heat. Add onion and sauté, stirring frequently until almost tender, about 15 minutes. Reduce heat to medium low and cook until nicely golden, stirring occasionally. Add wine and cook 4-5 minutes until evaporated.

2. Cook pasta according to package, leaving out oil and salt. Drain in a colander over a bowl to reserve ½ cup of the liquid. Add reserved liquid, pasta, radicchio, parsley, and oregano to the onion mixture. Add salt and pepper to taste, combine well, and top with cheese. Serve hot and enjoy!

Serves 4.

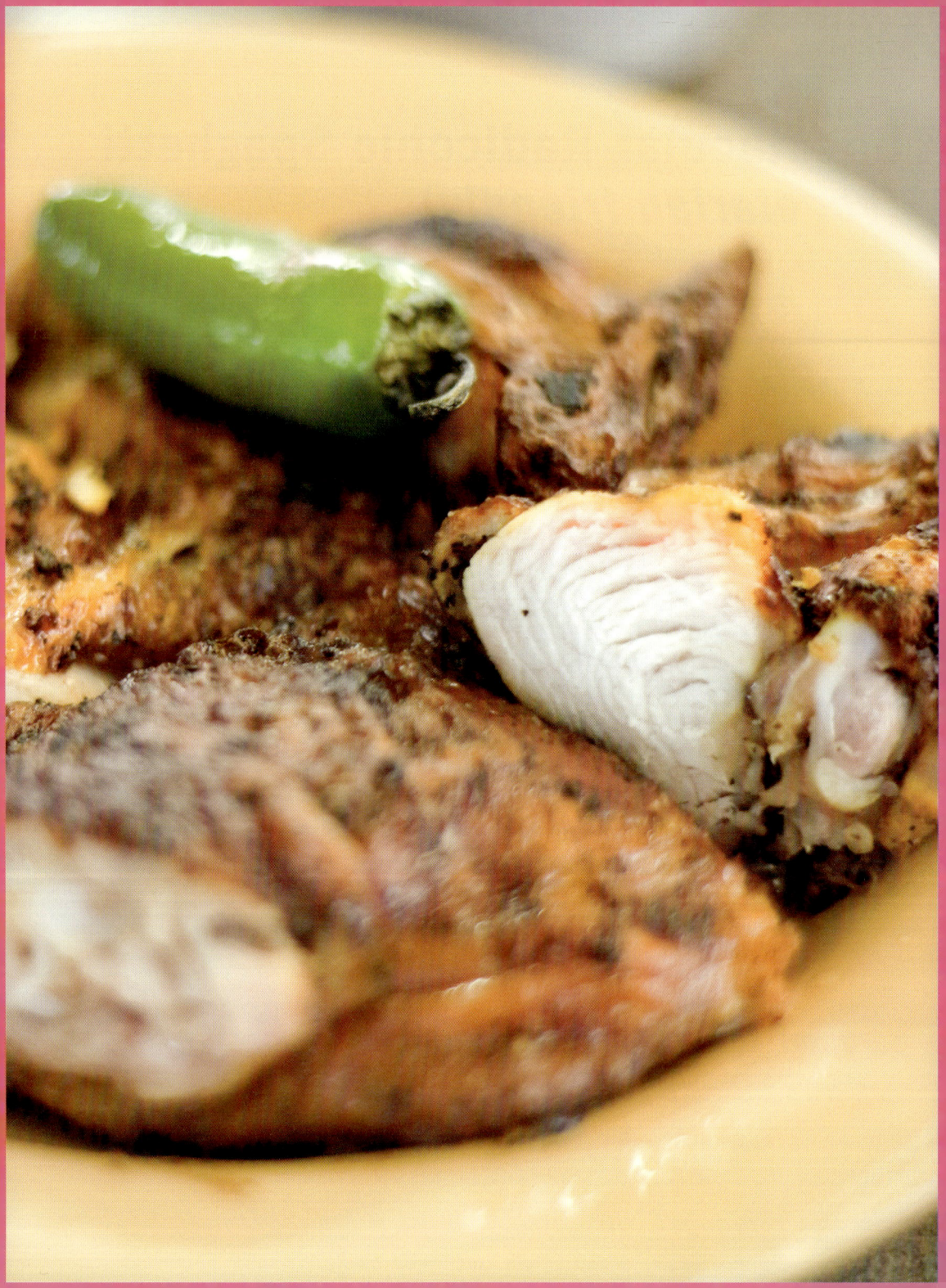

Jamaican Me Crazy Hot & Spicy Chicken

INGREDIENTS

½   tablespoon olive oil

½   cup minced red onion

1   tablespoon Truvia

1   tablespoon finely chopped jalapeño pepper (leave the seeds in if you want it hot!)

3   teaspoons cider vinegar

2   teaspoons low-sodium soy sauce (I like Kikkoman)

½   teaspoon salt

3/4   teaspoon ground allspice

3/4   teaspoon dried thyme

3/4   teaspoon freshly cracked black pepper

½   teaspoon cayenne

4   boneless skinless chicken breasts (trimmed)

    Fat-free cooking spray

DIRECTIONS

1. Combine olive oil through cayenne ingredients in a large bowl, add chicken, and toss to coat.

2. Coat a large skillet with non-fat cooking spray and heat on medium high. Add chicken and cook on both sides 4-5 minutes until browned and cooked through.

3. Serve hot with brown rice or a baked sweet potato, as the starchy side dish will cut the heat of the spice on the chicken. Enjoy!

Serves 4.

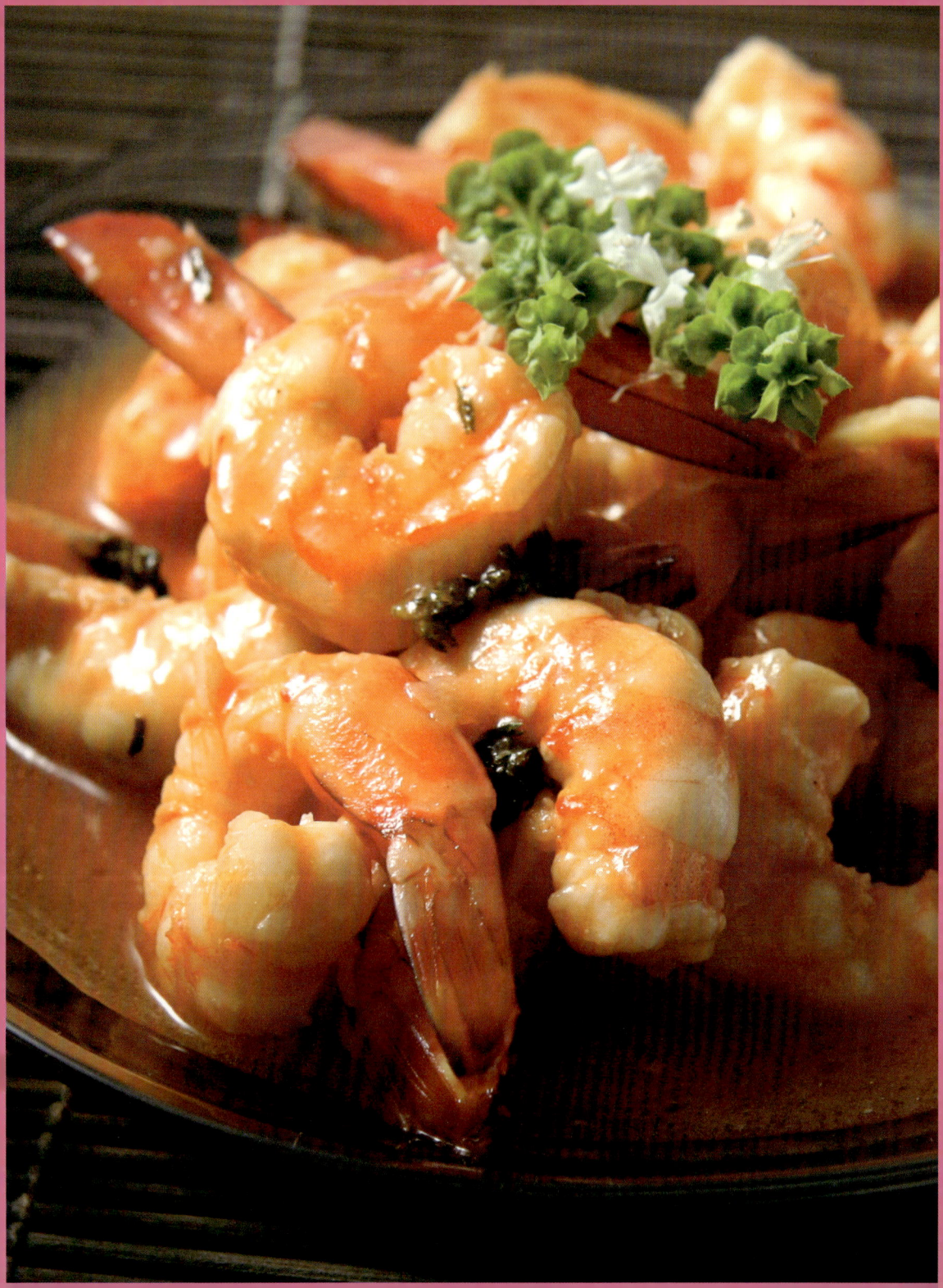

Spicy Brandied Shrimp with Rice

INGREDIENTS

2	tablespoons I Can't Believe It's Not Butter Light
¾	tablespoon olive oil
3	garlic cloves minced
1	pound shrimp, peeled and deveined
2 ½	teaspoons Worcestershire
¼	teaspoon Tabasco
	Salt

	Freshly ground black pepper
½	cup reduced-sugar ketchup
1 1/2	tablespoons chopped fresh oregano leaves
2 ½	tablespoons brandy
2 ½	tablespoons fresh flat leaf parsley, chopped

DIRECTIONS

1. Make rice according to package (I prefer converted brown in the husk for nutritional value).

2. Melt the butter with the olive oil in a large skillet over medium-high heat. Add garlic and stir for about 2 minutes. Stir in shrimp, Worcestershire, Tabasco, and salt and pepper to taste.

3. Simmer until shrimp are partially cooked, about 2 minutes.

4. Add reduced-sugar ketchup and oregano, stirring while simmering for about 2 more minutes, or until shrimp are opaque and cooked through. Add brandy and parsley, stirring to combine over heat for a quick 30 seconds.

5. Remove from heat and serve with rice. Enjoy!

Serves 2-4.

Hooray for Filet with Blue Cheese Crumbles

INGREDIENTS

¼ cup plain or whole wheat breadcrumbs

3 tablespoons reduced-fat blue cheese crumbles

2 ½ teaspoons fines herbes

½ teaspoon olive oil
Fat-free cooking spray, olive oil flavor

4 6-ounce filet mignon steaks

1 teaspoon freshly cracked black pepper

½ cup red wine or cognac

1 cup reduced-sodium beef broth

½ cup chopped sweet onion

1 teaspoon minced garlic
Salt
Pepper

DIRECTIONS

1. Line a baking sheet with foil and preheat oven to 400 degrees.

2. In a small bowl, combine breadcrumbs, blue cheese, fines herbes, and olive oil. Coat a large skillet with fat-free cooking spray and heat over medium high heat.

3. Season the steaks with pepper to taste, about ½ teaspoon total, and add to skillet, cooking for about 2 minutes per side. Remove steaks from skillet and transfer to the prepared baking sheet, topping each with ¼ of the blue cheese mixture. Cook in oven 4-6 minutes until cooked to taste (about 4 minutes for medium rare and 5-6 minutes for medium).

TO MAKE THE SAUCE

1. Return the steak skillet to the heat and pour in the red wine or cognac. Add reduced-sodium beef broth, onions, and garlic.

2. Bring mixture to a boil and cook until it thickens and reduces.

3. Strain the sauce into a gravy boat, removing large chunks, and distribute evenly over the steaks. Season steaks with salt and pepper to taste and serve hot.

Serves 4.

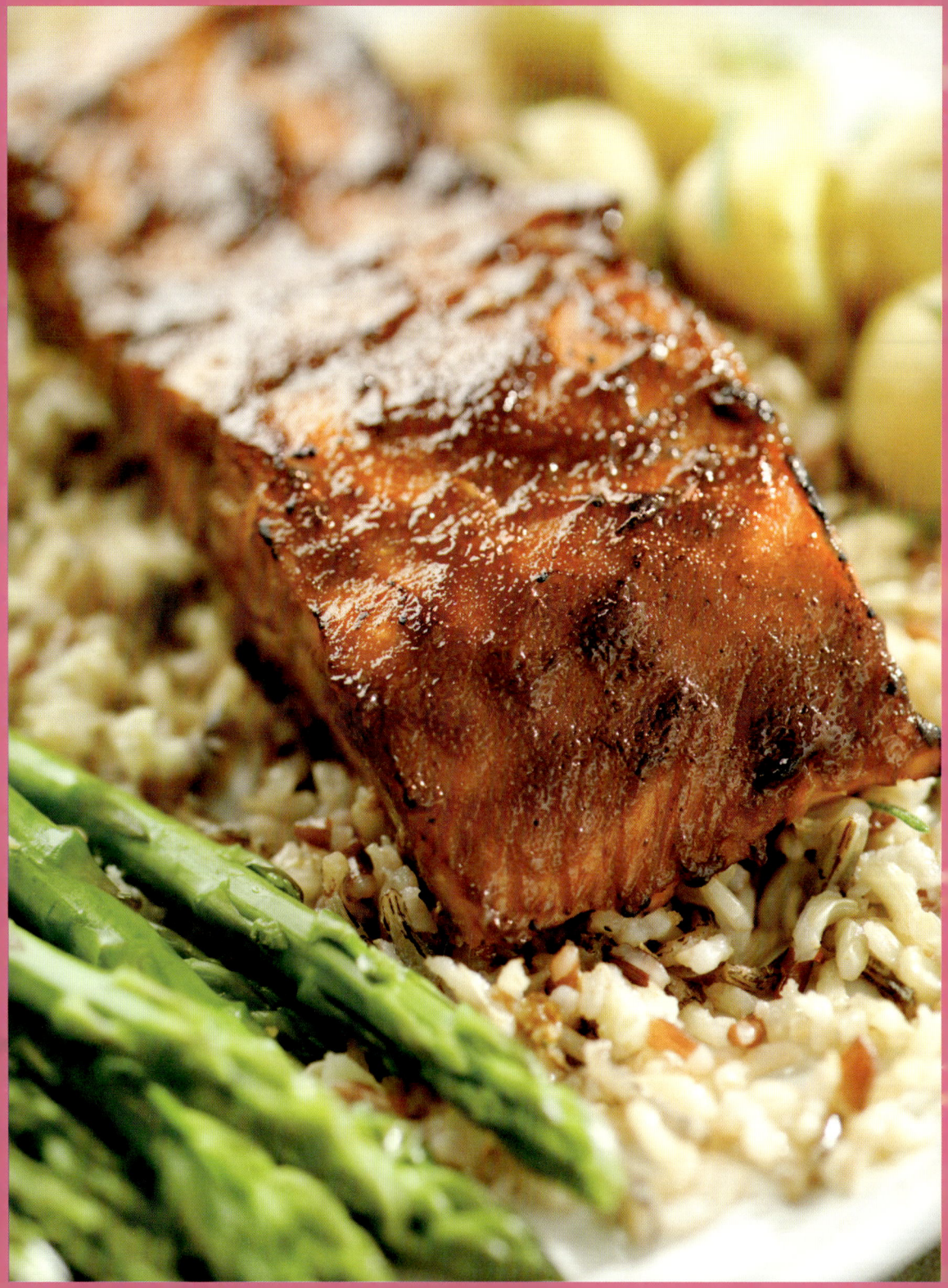

Orange & Ginger Smothered Salmon with Rice

INGREDIENTS

1 ½	pounds salmon (4 serving size filets)
¾	cup reduced-sugar orange juice
½	cup all-fruit orange marmalade
1	tablespoon Dijon mustard
2	teaspoons citrus herb seasoning
1 ½	teaspoons minced ginger

DIRECTIONS

1. Prepare rice as directed. Line a baking sheet with foil and set aside. Prepare salmon by rinsing, patting dry, and placing in a plastic bag.

2. In a small bowl, combine reduced-sugar orange juice, marmalade, mustard citrus herb seasoning, and ginger. Pour into plastic bag with the salmon, let out excess air, seal, and mix ingredients in bag to coat salmon. Refrigerate for 2 hours.

3. Remove fish from fridge 15 to 20 minutes prior to turning on broiler. Turn on broiler and preheat for 5 minutes. Transfer salmon to prepared baking sheet and broil about 6 inches from heat for 4-6 minutes per side. Salmon should flake easily with a fork when done.

4. Serve hot with a side of converted brown rice in the husk (for lunch) or steamed asparagus (this is the dinnertime, no-starch version) and enjoy!

Serves 4.

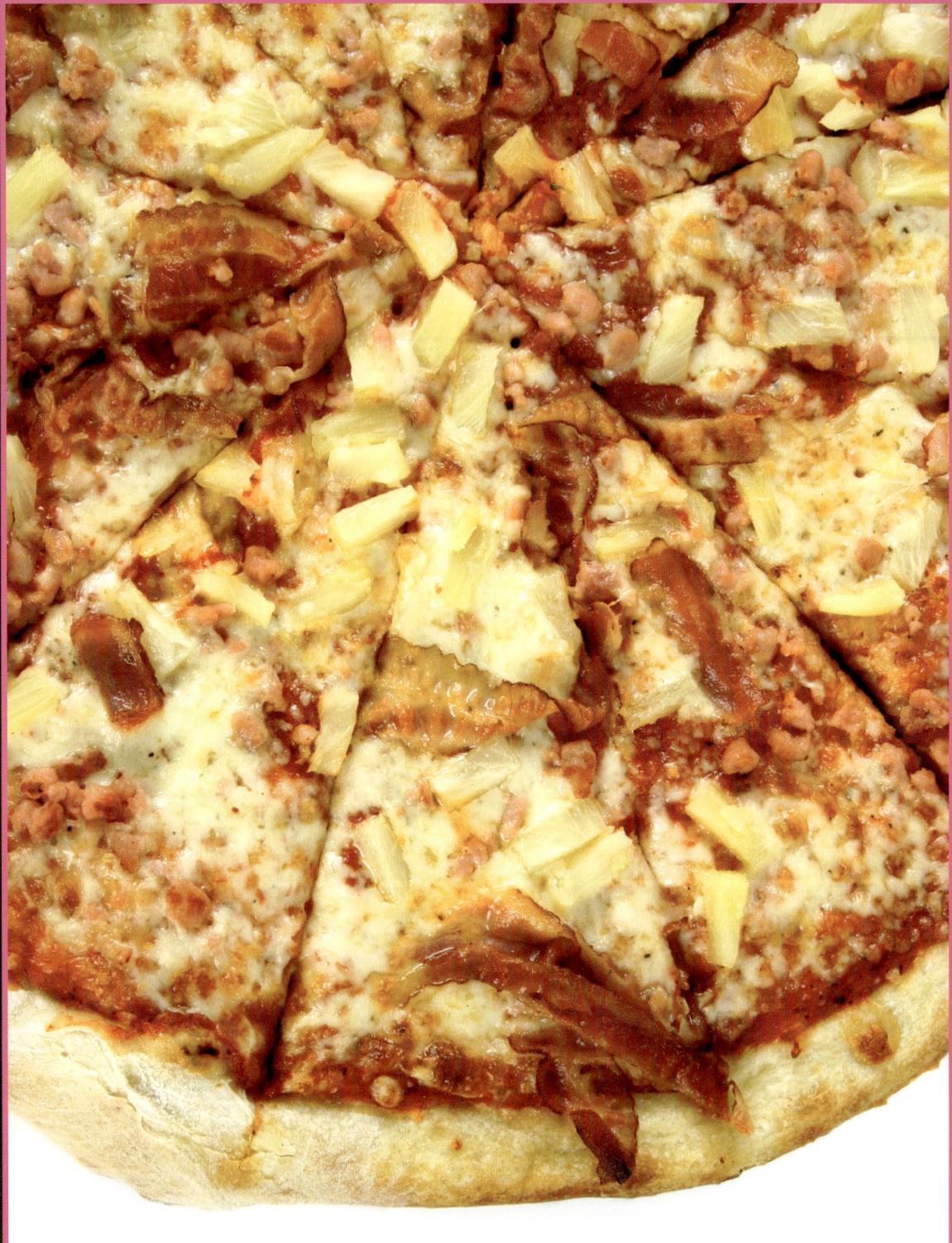

Simply Sinless Canadian Bacon Pizza

INGREDIENTS

1	whole wheat pizza crust
¼	cup reduced-fat blue cheese salad dressing
1	cup reduced-fat mozzarella cheese
3/4	cup chopped pineapple (canned is easiest)
3	tablespoons pineapple juice (from the above can)
½	cup chopped sweet onion
½	cup chopped Canadian bacon (leaner ham may be used to save more calories) Reduced-fat grated Parmesan to taste

DIRECTIONS

1. Preheat oven according to directions on crust. I prefer to bake directly on the rack for a crispier crust, but a baking sheet may also be used.

2. In a medium bowl, combine salad dressing, cheese, and pineapple juice. Mix well and spread onto pizza crust. Top pizza with pineapple, onion, and Canadian bacon or ham.

3. Bake in preheated oven for 12-17 minutes or until crust is golden brown. Top with reduced-fat grated Parmesan to taste and serve hot.

Serves 4.

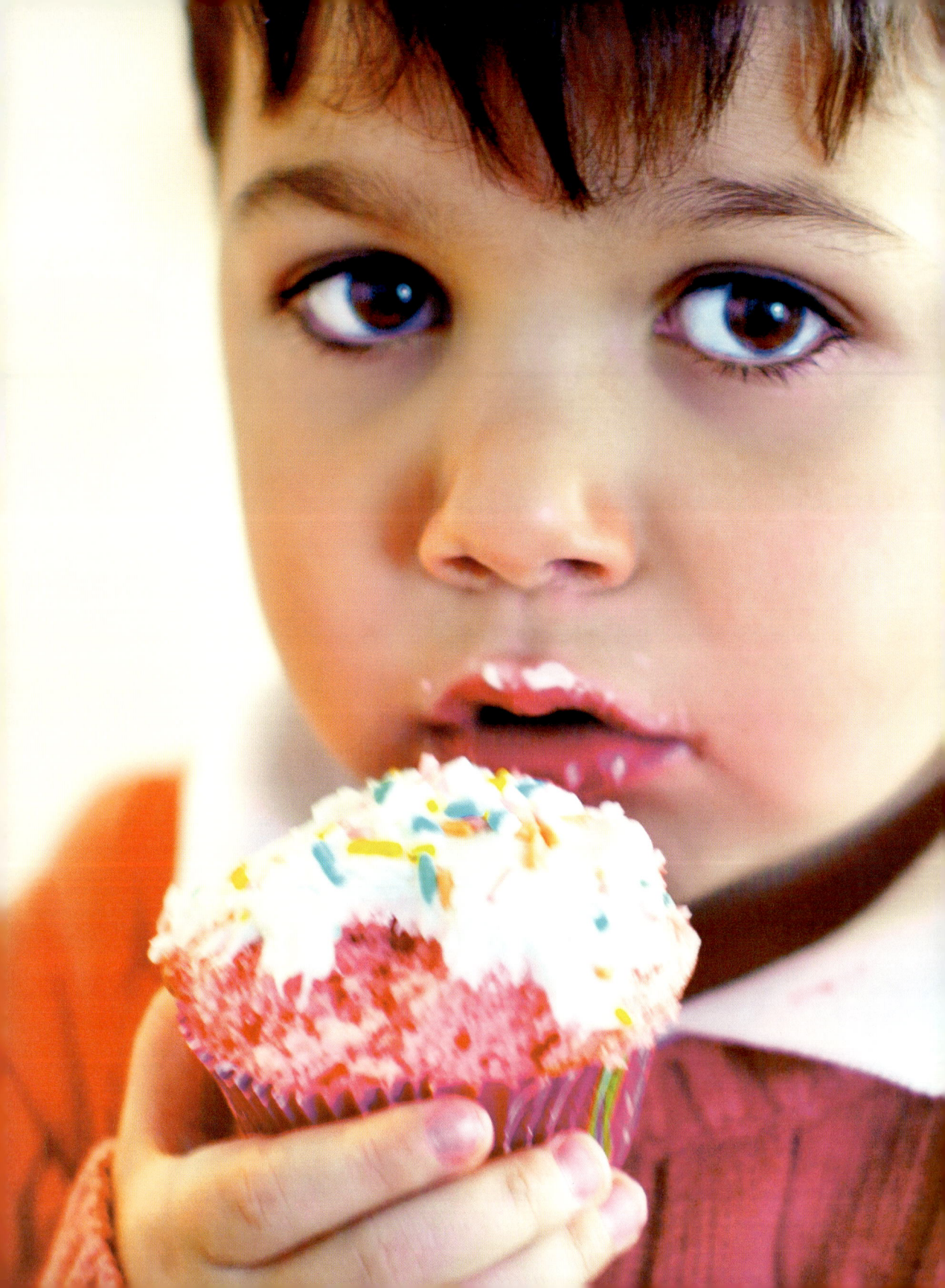

Chapter 10 :

Simply Sinless Desserts

Yes, you can have dessert! Remember that we now do everything in moderation, including moderation! Making wise decisions all day leaves room for a little treat, and as with the other recipes, these are light and yummy. In fact, some are Simply Sinless, so enjoy!

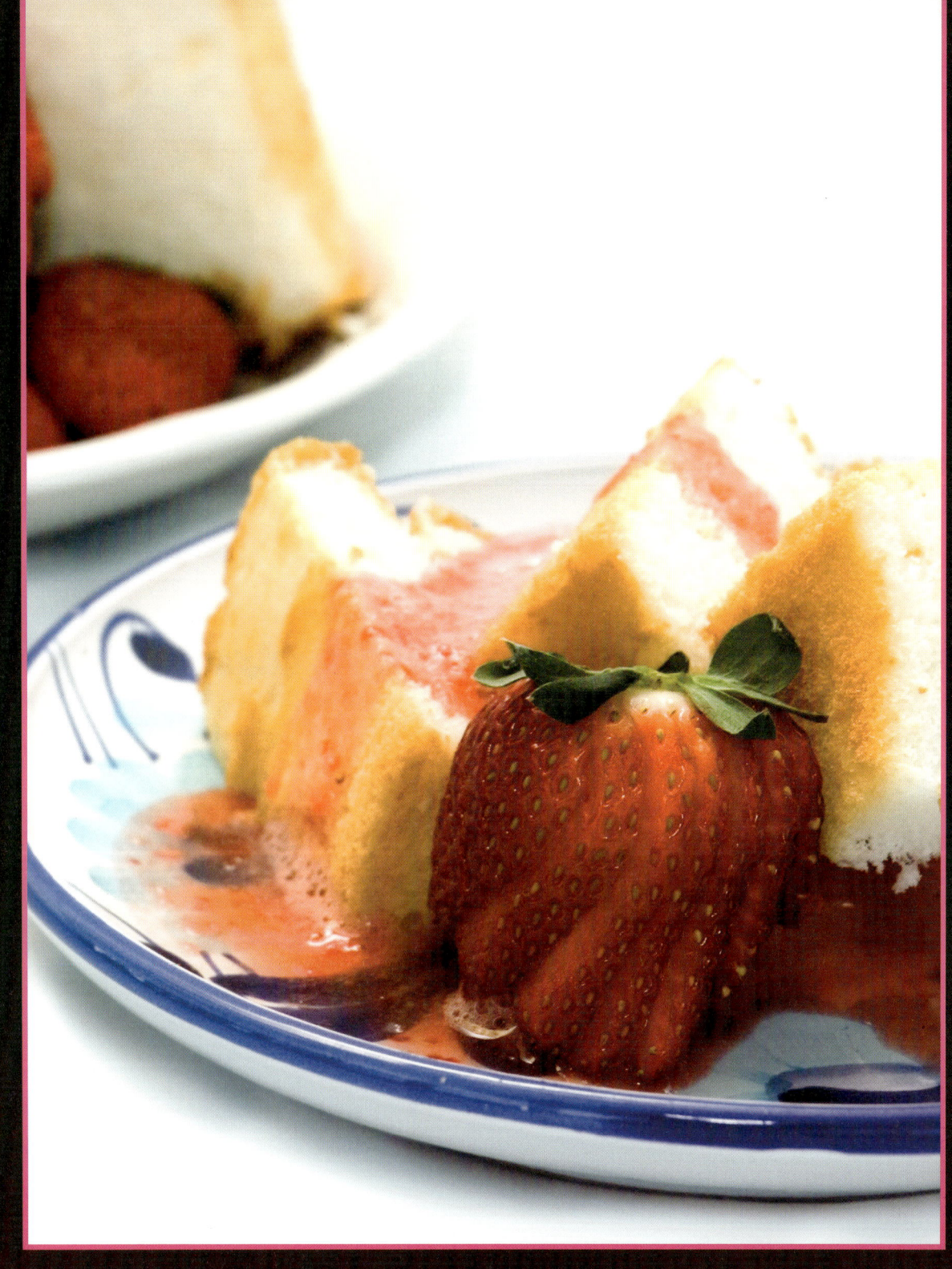

Simply Sinless Aren't You an Angelfood Cake with Berries

INGREDIENTS

1 store-bought reduced-fat angel food cake (this also comes in a sugar-free variety)

1 bag previously frozen strawberries, no sugar added

1 12-ounce container fresh blueberries

1 12-ounce container fresh raspberries

2 tablespoons water

Truvia to taste (I usually use about ½ cup)

Reddi Whip Light, optional

DIRECTIONS

1. Rinse and drain blueberries and raspberries and combine in a medium bowl with previously frozen strawberries. Add 2 tablespoons water and mix well with a wooden spoon. Press firmly on some of the strawberries to soften them and make them somewhat mushy. Add ½ cup Truvia and mix until thoroughly blended. Taste for sweetness. Some prefer this a little sweeter, so add more Truvia if needed.

2. Cut angel food cake into serving pieces and place in dishes or in small bowls. Drizzle fruit mixture evenly over each piece. Sprinkle a little Truvia on top, add Reddi Whip Light, and serve!

Serves 8-10.

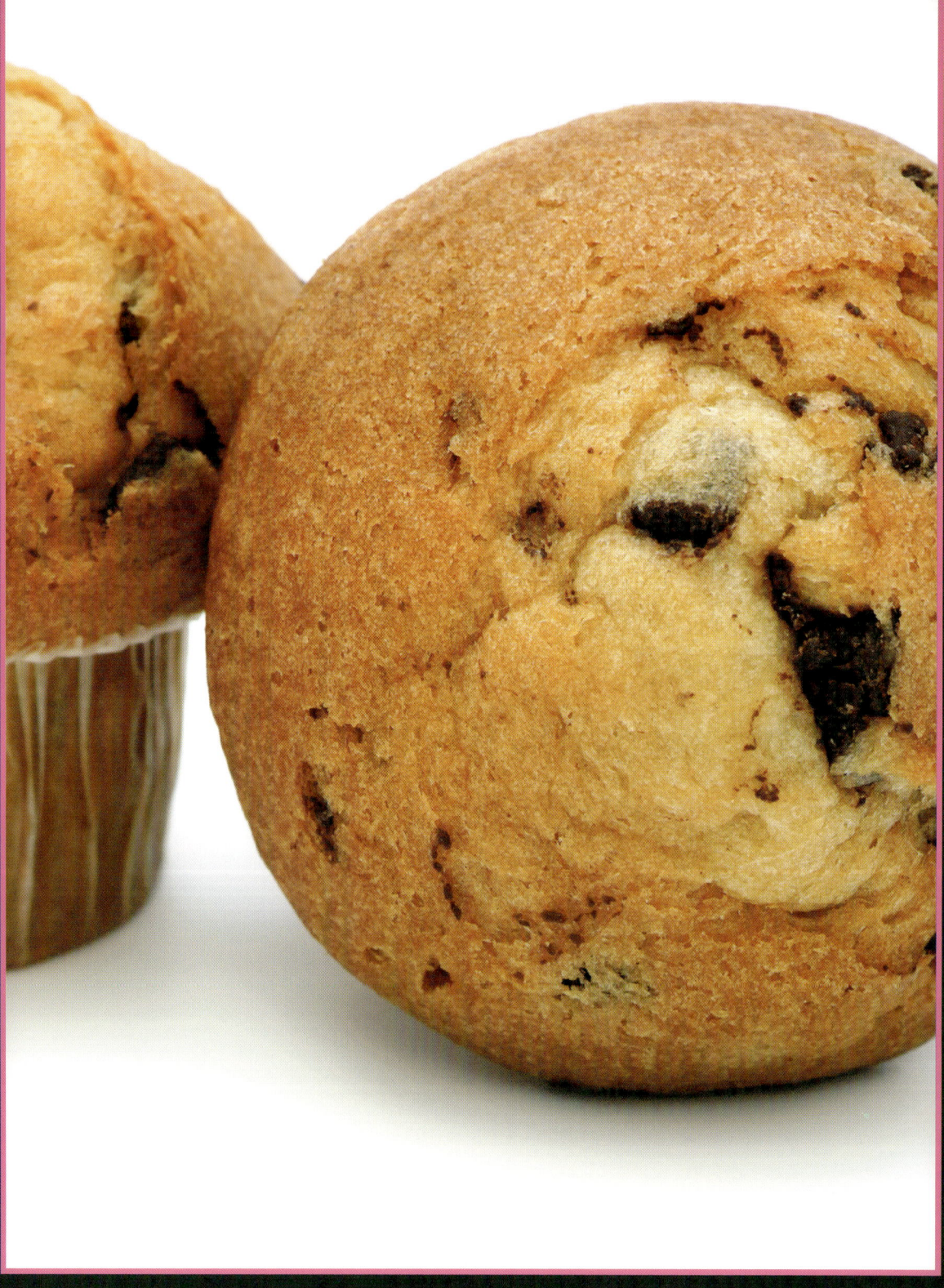

Banana Chocolate Chip Muffins

INGREDIENTS

1 cup all-purpose flour	½ cup Splenda Brown Sugar Blend
1 cup whole wheat four	2 tablespoons no sugar added applesauce
½ cup rolled oats	2 teaspoons vegetable oil
2 teaspoons ground cinnamon	2 large egg whites
2 teaspoons baking powder	1 large egg
1 teaspoon baking soda	1 ¼ cups reduced-fat buttermilk
½ teaspoon salt	1 teaspoon pure vanilla extract
1 large ripe banana, mashed	2 tablespoons milk or dark chocolate chips
¼ cup chopped pecans or walnuts	

DIRECTIONS

1. Preheat oven to 400 degrees. Line a 12-muffin muffin tray with festive liners and set aside.

2. In mixer, combine both flours, rolled oats, cinnamon, baking powder, baking soda, salt, and mashed banana and blend on low for 2 minutes. Add nuts, Splenda, applesauce, vegetable oil, egg whites, egg, and reduced-fat buttermilk and blend for another 2 minutes on medium speed. Add vanilla and mix until well blended.

3. Using a ¼-cup measuring cup, portion the batter evenly into the muffin cups and top each muffin with 4-5 chocolate chips. Bake at 400 degrees for 15 minutes. Once golden and baked through, remove from oven and serve warm.

Makes 12 muffins.

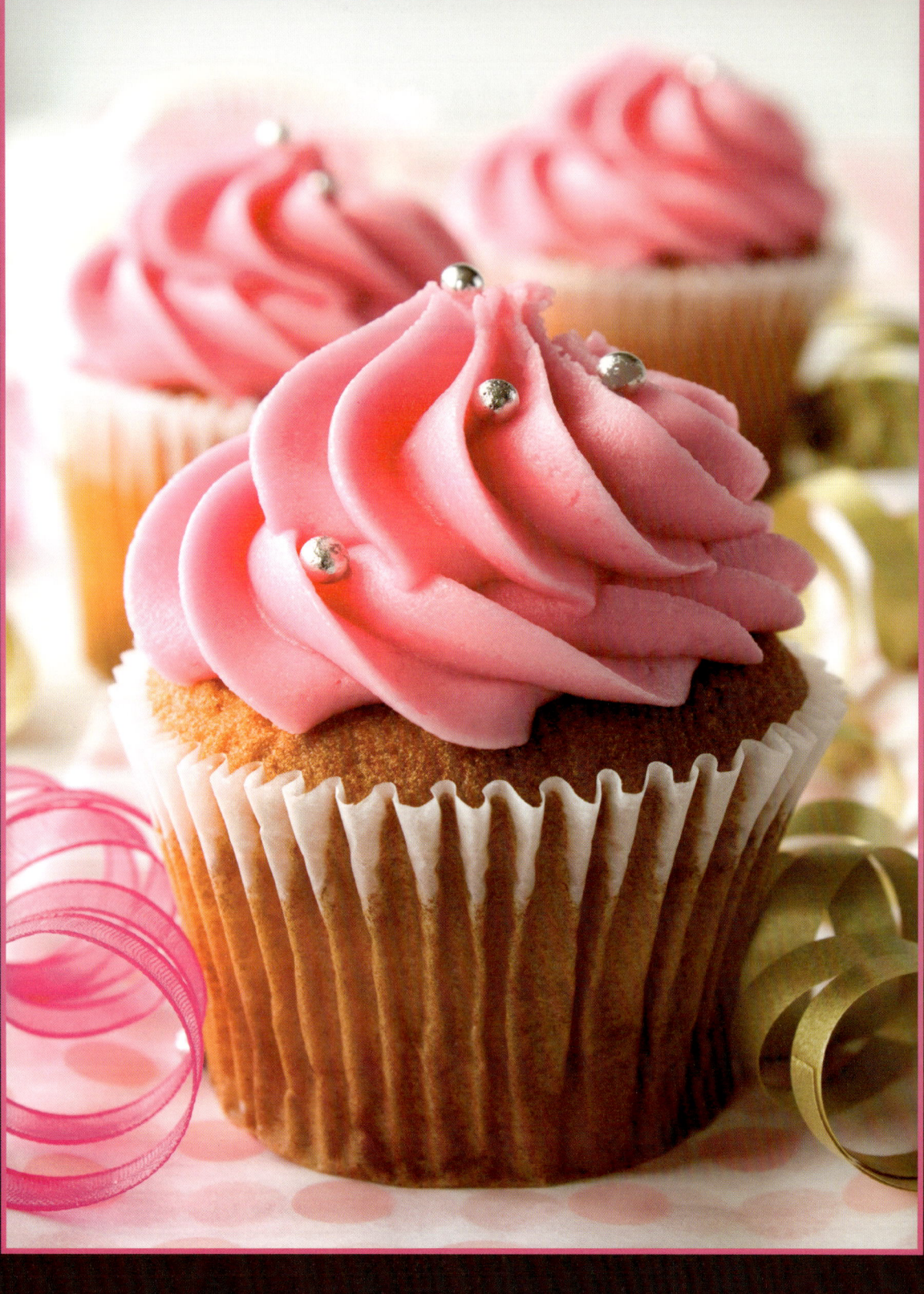

Va-Va Vanilla Cupcakes

INGREDIENTS

1 ¼   cups all-purpose flour
½   cup finely ground almonds
1 ½   teaspoons baking powder
¼   teaspoon salt
2   large egg whites

1   large egg
½   cup Truvia
2   teaspoons pure vanilla extract
1 ¼   cups peeled zucchini, finely grated

INGREDIENTS FOR FROSTING

3   large egg whites
¾   cup Truvia
       Pinch of salt
¾   teaspoon pure vanilla extract

Zest of ½ lemon
Food coloring optional for colored frosting
Sprinkles, decorations optional

DIRECTIONS

1. Preheat the oven to 350 degrees and line a 12-muffin muffin pan with festive liners.

2. In a bowl, whisk together flour, almonds, and baking powder. In a second bowl, beat the egg whites, egg, Truvia, salt, and vanilla until thickened, about 4 minutes. Beat in the zucchini until well blended.

3. Slowly add the dry ingredients and beat on low until well blended. Use a 1/3-cup measuring cup to scoop and pour evenly into muffin pan. Bake in preheated oven 20-25 minutes or until inserted toothpick comes out clean.

4. As cupcakes bake, make the frosting by combining egg whites, Truvia, salt, and vanilla extract in a heatproof bowl over a pan of simmering water. Stir continuously 1-2 minutes over heat until mixture is warm and Truvia has dissolved.

5. Remove bowl from heat and beat mixture on high until it has cooled entirely and stiffens, about 6-7 minutes. Add lemon zest and beat until smooth. Let frosting cool in the refrigerator about 30 minutes.

6. Once cupcakes have baked, remove and cool completely before frosting. Serve and enjoy!

Makes 12 muffins.

Perfect Peanut Butter Crumb Cake

INGREDIENTS

1   package yellow cake mix
¾   cup reduced-fat peanut butter
¼   cup Splenda Brown Sugar
      Baking Blend
1   cup water
¾   cup egg whites

¼   cup sugar-free applesauce
1   tablespoon vegetable oil
1/3   cup mini chocolate chips (semi-
         sweet or milk chocolate)
¼   cup peanut butter chips
¼   cup roasted peanuts, finely chopped

DIRECTIONS

1. Preheat oven to 350 degrees and spray 13 x 9-inch baking pan with fat-free cooking spray.

2. In a large bowl, beat the cake mix, peanut butter, and Splenda on low until mixture is crumbly. Separate 1/3 cup of the mixture and set aside in another bowl for topping. In the main bowl, add water, egg whites, applesauce, and oil and beat on medium speed until well blended.

3. Spread batter evenly in the prepared pan. In the topping bowl, add chocolate chips, peanut butter chips, and peanuts and mix well. Sprinkle the mixture over the batter in the pan.

4. Bake 38-40 minutes or until inserted toothpick comes out clean. Cool on a wire rack, serve, and enjoy!

Serves 8-10.

Three Layers of Heaven Chocolate Cream Cloud

INGREDIENTS FOR CRUST

1 ¼   cups all-purpose flour
¼   cup powdered sugar
6   tablespoons I Can't Believe It's
     Not Butter Light

¼   cup toasted pecans, finely chopped
     Fat-free cooking spray, butter flavored

INGREDIENTS FOR FILLING

1   cup Splenda
½   cup reduced-fat cream
     cheese, softened
½   cup fat-free cream
     cheese, softened
1   carton Cool Whip Light,
     thawed and divided

3   cups 1% low-fat milk
2   3.9-ounce packages Sugar-Free Jell-O
     Instant Chocolate Pudding
     Nestle unsweetened cocoa
      for sprinkling

DIRECTIONS

1. Preheat oven to 325 degrees.

2. For crust, spoon flour into measuring cups and level. In a medium bowl, combine flour with ¼ cup Splenda and stir together gently until well blended. Add butter and beat on low until well blended and coarse. Stir in pecans and press firmly into a 13 x 9-inch prepared baking pan. Bake at 325 degrees for 18-20 minutes until lightly browned.

3. For filling, in medium bowl, beat 1 cup Splenda and cream cheeses at medium speed until fluffy. Fold in ½ of the Cool Whip Light. Spread mixture over the cooled crust, cover with plastic wrap, and chill for 1 hour.

4. Combine milk and pudding in a large bowl, mixing at medium speed for about 2 minutes. Cover and chill for about 1 hour or until it sets. After it sets, spread pudding mixture over cream cheese layer. Spread remaining ½ of Cool Whip Light on top as the third layer and cover and chill for another 30 minutes to set.

5. Sprinkle with cocoa and serve chilled.

Serves 12 or more.

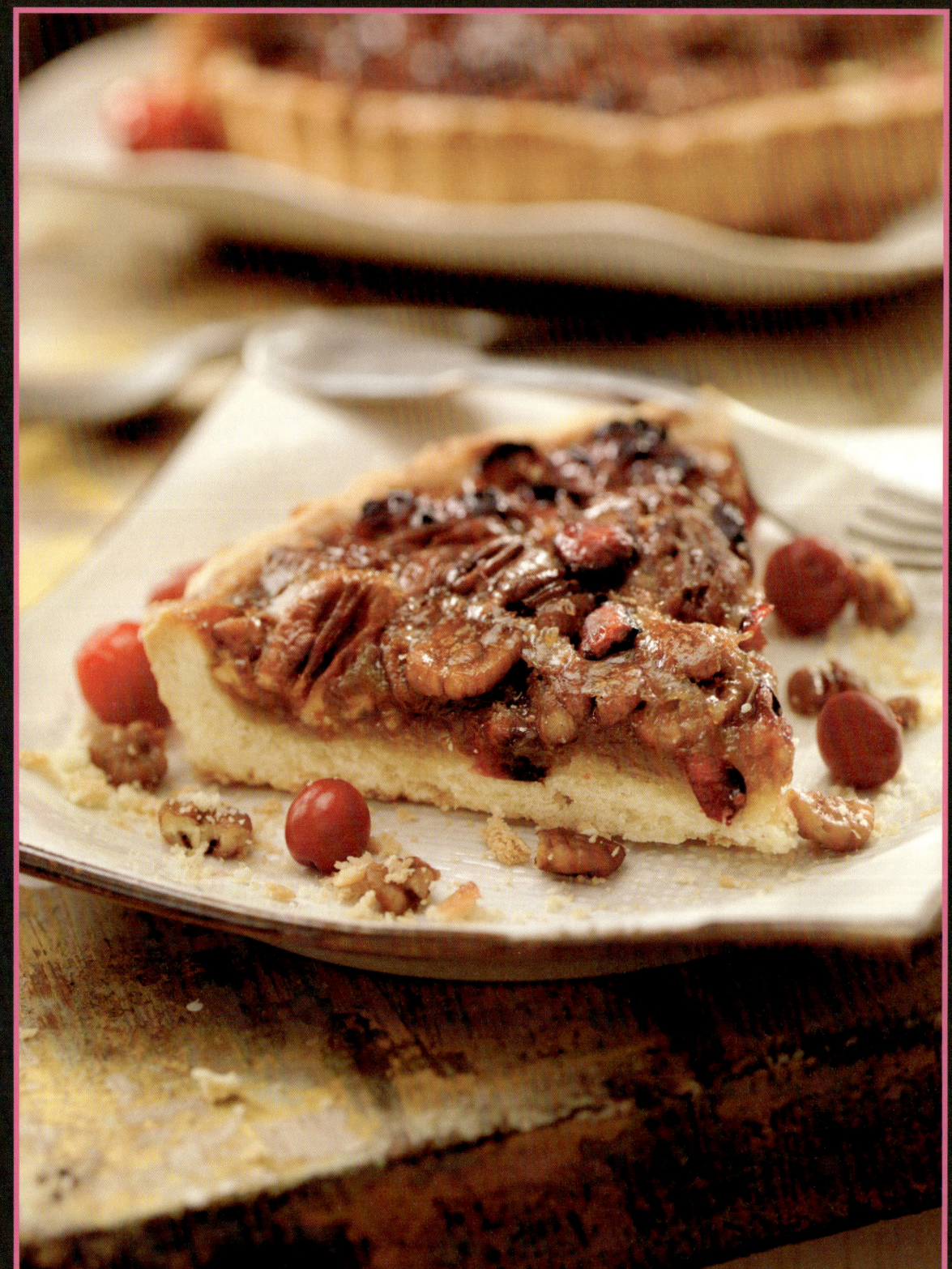

Simply Sinless White Chocolate Berry Tartlet

INGREDIENTS

1 refrigerated pie crust

¾ cup Truvia

2 egg whites

1 egg

¼ cup I Can't Believe It's Not Butter Light, melted

2 teaspoons pure vanilla extract

½ cup all-purpose flour

6 1-ounce squares white chocolate, chopped

½ cup chopped, lightly toasted macadamia nuts or pecans

½ cup dried cranberries or cherries, chopped

DIRECTIONS

1. Preheat oven to 350 degrees and place pie crust in 9-inch pie pan.

2. In a large bowl, combine Truvia, egg whites, egg, melted butter, and vanilla.

3. Mix well. Stir in flour until well blended. Add white chocolate, nuts, and cranberries and stir until well blended.

4. Pour filling into unbaked crust and bake 50-55 minutes or until the top is golden brown and an inserted knife comes out clean. Cool completely on a wire rack.

Makes 6 generous servings, or 8 smaller ones.

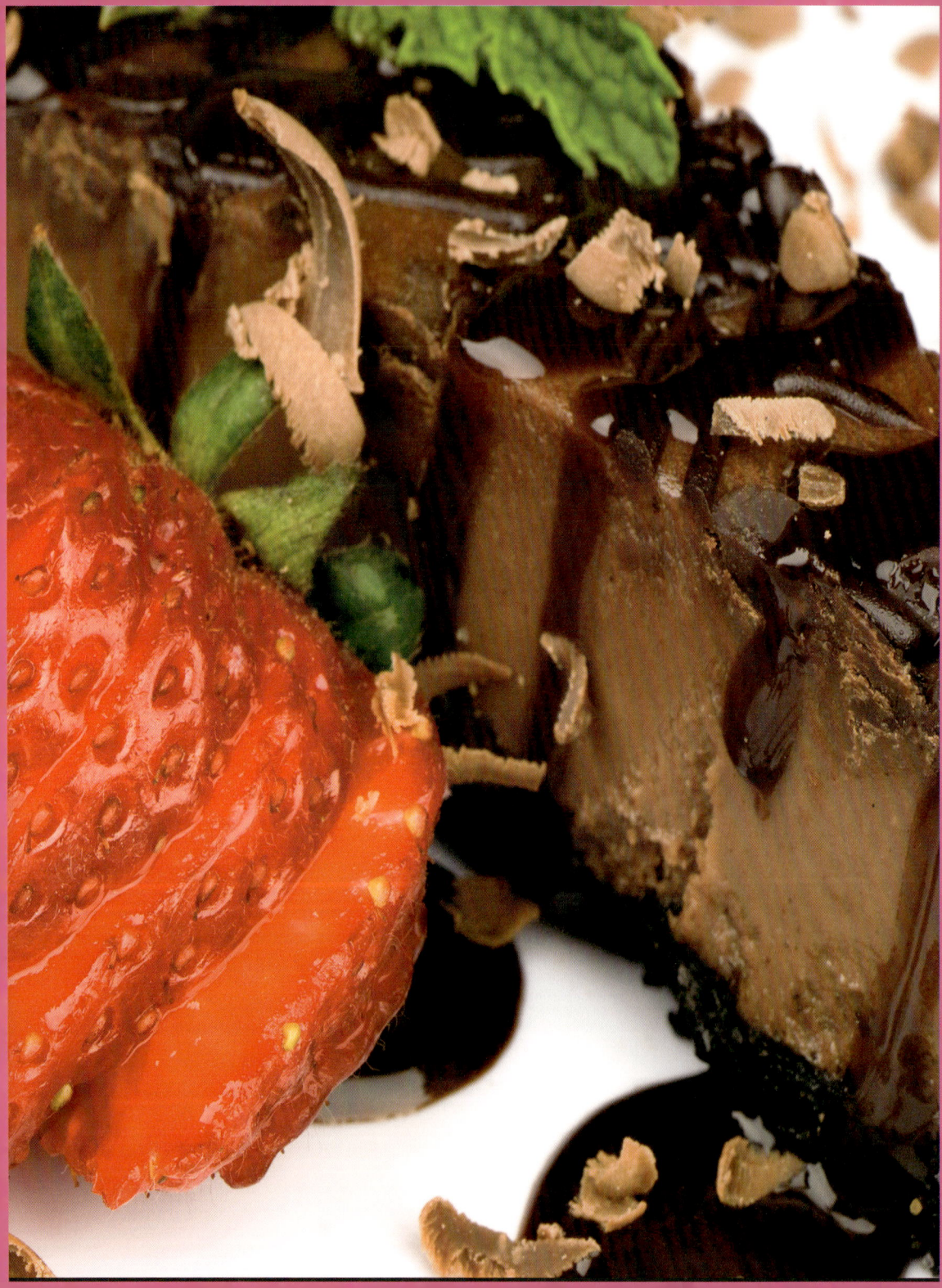

Simply Sinless No-Bake Chocolate Cheesecake

INGREDIENTS

1 8-ounce semi-sweet chocolate baking bar, melted and cooled

2 8-ounce packages reduced-fat cream cheese, softened

¾ cup Splenda Brown Sugar Baking Blend

¼ cup Splenda

2 tablespoons 1% milk

1 teaspoon pure vanilla extract

1 prepared 9-inch chocolate crumb crust

Reddi Whip Light, optional

Sliced strawberries for garnish

DIRECTIONS

1. In a medium bowl, beat the cream cheese, both Splenda blends, and vanilla extract on high for about 2 minutes, until well blended. Add melted chocolate and beat on medium speed for another 2 minutes.

2. Spoon into crust and refrigerate until set, about an hour or so. Top with Reddi Whip Light and serve.

Serves 6-8.

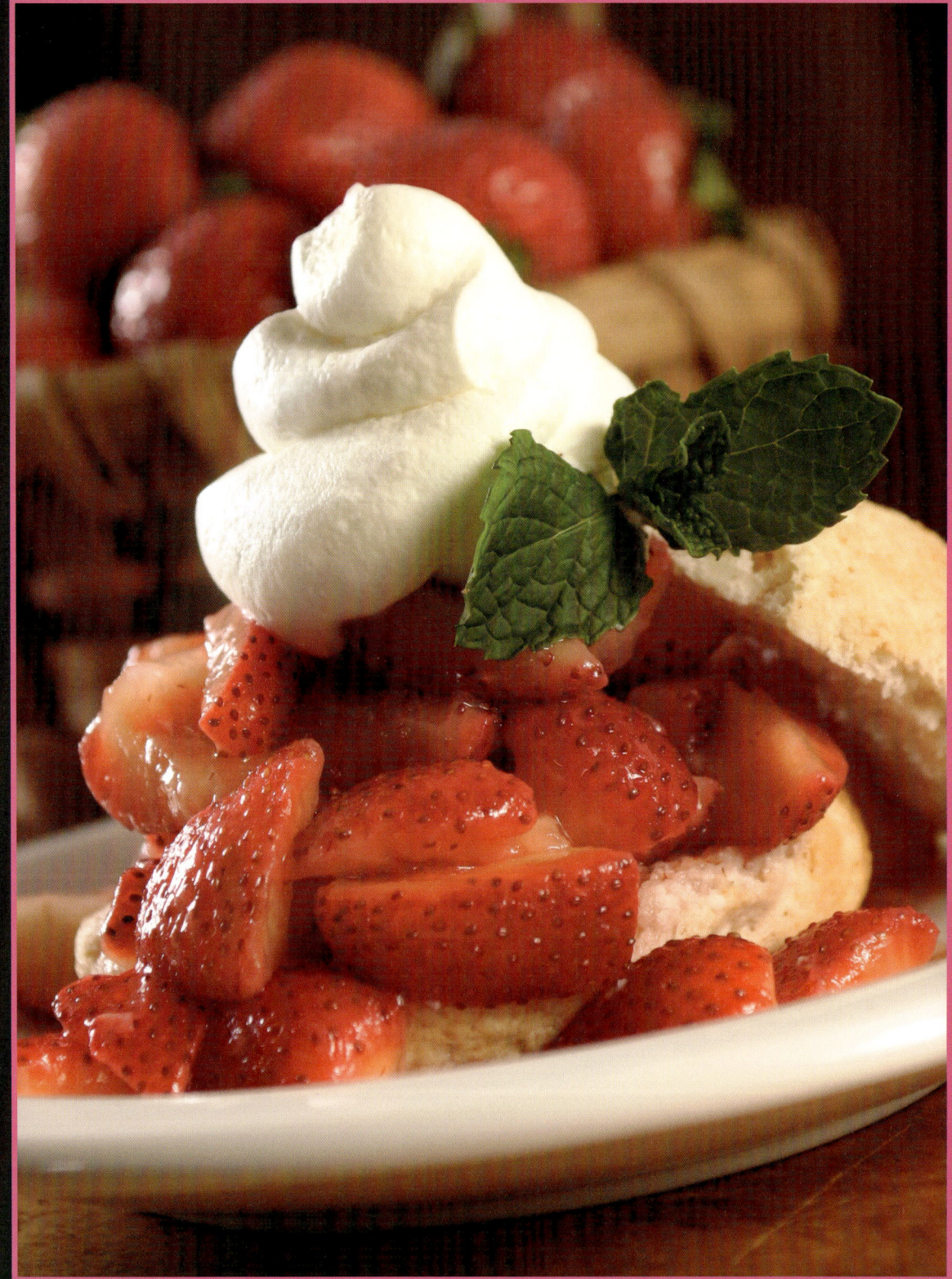

Simply Sinless Strawberry Shortcake

INGREDIENTS

3   baskets of fresh strawberries (consider adding 1 3-6-ounce container of blueberries, too, as they're a great source of antioxidants)

1/2   cup Splenda or Truvia
1/4   cup water
1   can Reddi Whip Light or Reddi Whip Fat Free (with the light blue top)

DIRECTIONS

1. Remove the stems from the strawberries and slice thinly, then pour into a large bowl. Mix in blueberries, if using. Add 1/4 cup-1/2 cup Splenda or Truvia (depending on how sweet the strawberries are to begin with) and mix into the strawberries. Add 1/4 cup water and mix well. Place in fridge to chill.

2. After the strawberries have been chilling for 20 minutes or so, take a potato masher and mash them a little. Not too much, just enough to get juice out of them. Place the strawberries back in the fridge and continue chilling as you make the biscuits.

INGREDIENTS FOR BISCUITS

2 1/3   cups Bisquick baking mix
3   tablespoons I Can't Believe It's Not Butter Light, melted

1/2   cup 1% milk
3   tablespoons Splenda or Truvia

        fat-free cooking spray

DIRECTIONS

1. Heat oven to 425°F and spray cookie sheet with cooking spray.

2. Stir Bisquick mix, melted butter, reduced-fat milk, and Splenda or Truvia in a mixing bowl until soft dough forms.

3. Drop 6 spoonfuls onto the prepared cookie sheet. Bake 10-12 minutes or until golden brown.

TO MAKE THE DESSERT

1. Slice biscuits in half and place in bowls, then gently spoon even amounts of chilled strawberry/blueberry mixture over the biscuits.

2. Add a spray of fat-free Reddi Whip to each bowl, serve immediately, and enjoy!

Serves 6.

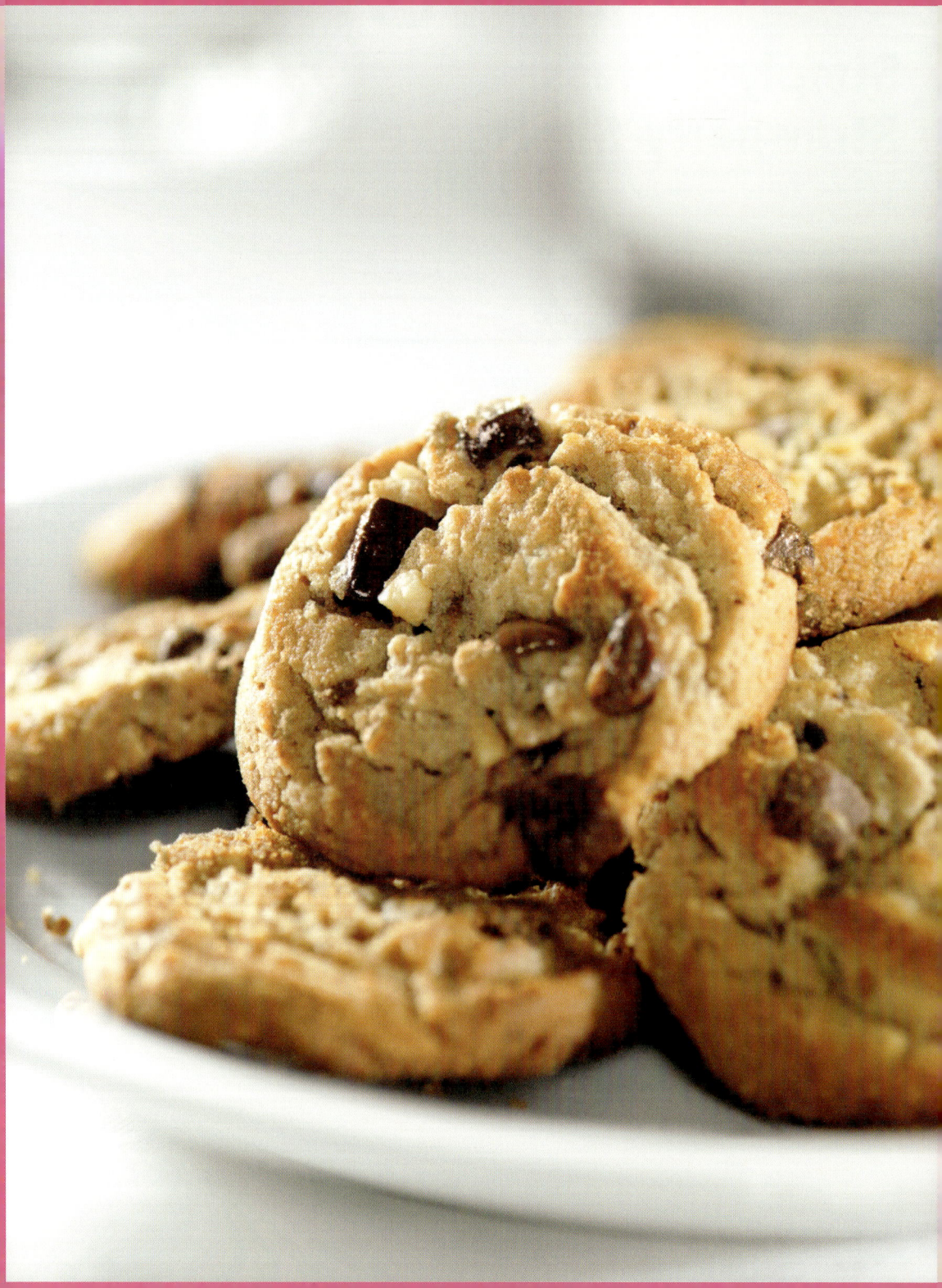

Chocolate Peanut Butter Favorite Cookies

These cookies are the healthier version of a yummy favorite. Moderation is key. Don't eat a dozen, but two or three won't blow your calorie budget.

INGREDIENTS

1/2	cup I Can't Believe It's Not Butter Light, softened	2	egg whites (or 2 eggs if you prefer a heavier cookie)
		1	teaspoon vanilla extract
1/2	cup reduced-fat creamy or chunky peanut butter	1 1/2	cups all-purpose flour
		1/2	teaspoon baking soda
1/2	cup Splenda	1/4	teaspoon salt
1/2	cup Splenda Brown Sugar Blend	1	cup milk chocolate morsels

DIRECTIONS

1. Heat oven to 350 degrees and spray cookie sheet with nonfat cooking spray.

2. Beat softened butter and peanut butter in a large bowl on medium until well mixed and creamy in texture. Slowly add Splenda and Splenda Brown Sugar Blend, beating until mixed thoroughly. Add egg whites (or eggs) and vanilla and beat until almost fluffy.

3. In a separate bowl, mix flour, baking soda, and salt with a whisk until well combined. Slowly pour the flour mixture into the peanut butter mixture and beat on low until well blended. Stir in 1 cup of milk chocolate morsels (you can add another half cup if you prefer a more chocolaty taste) until well combined.

4. Drop by rounded tablespoons onto prepared cookie sheet.

5. Bake at 350 degrees for 10-12 minutes until lightly browned and edges appear a hint crispy. Remove from sheet to wire baking racks to cool.

Makes 24 cookies.

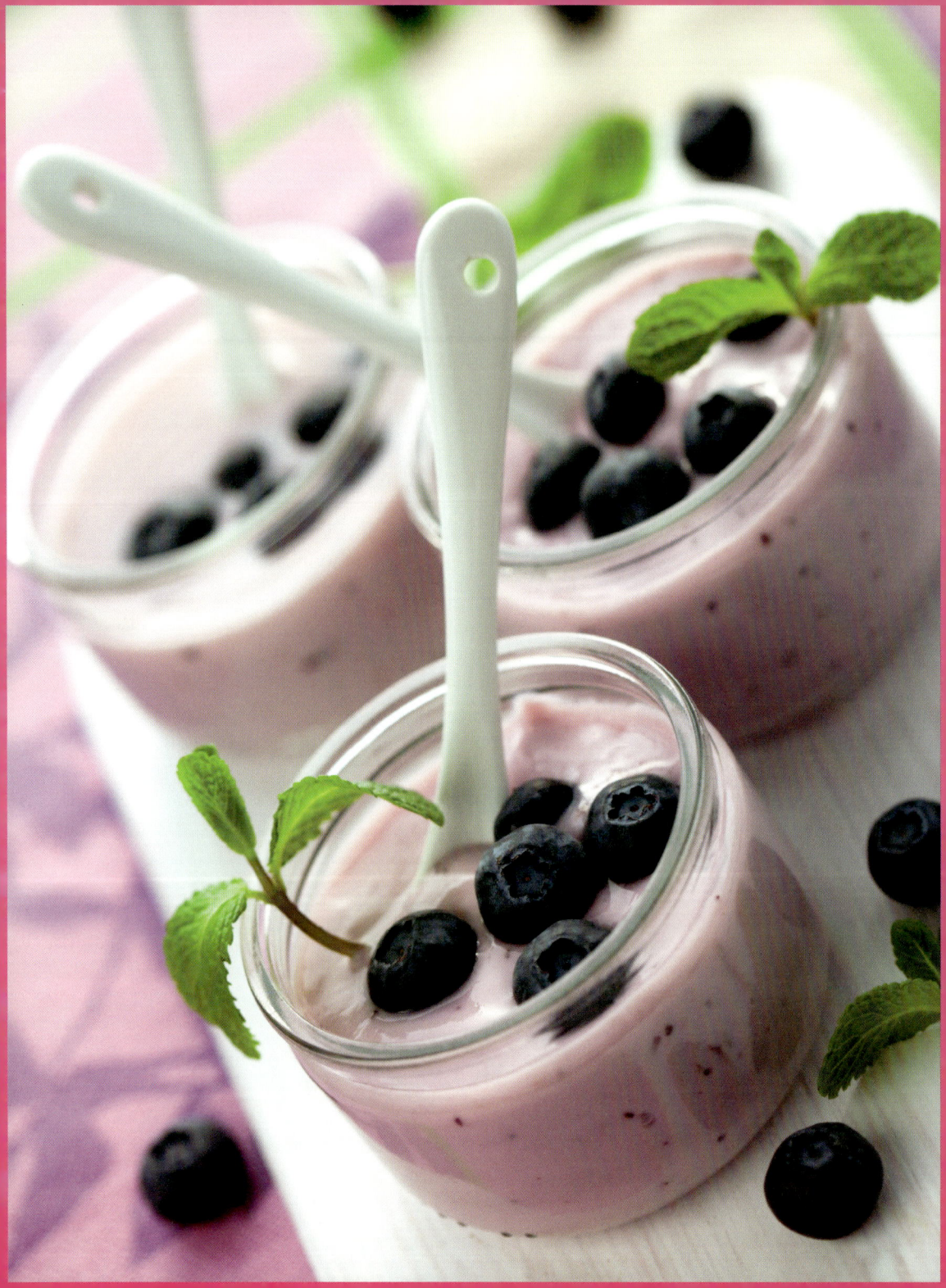

Simply Sinless Black & Blue Great Greek Yogurt

INGREDIENTS

2/3 cup frozen blueberries

2/3 cup frozen blackberries

½ cup water

½ cup Splenda or Truvia

2 tablespoons fresh lemon juice

1 tablespoon I Can't Believe It's Not Butter Light

2 cups plain fat-free or low-fat Greek yogurt

Garnish with blackberries

DIRECTIONS

1. Combine first 5 ingredients in a small saucepan and bring to a boil. Reduce heat to medium low and simmer for 10 minutes until thickened. Stir in butter.

2. Spoon ½ cup yogurt into 4 bowls and top each serving with ¼ cup of the sauce, stirring into the yogurt or leave as a topping. Serve immediately.

Serves 4.

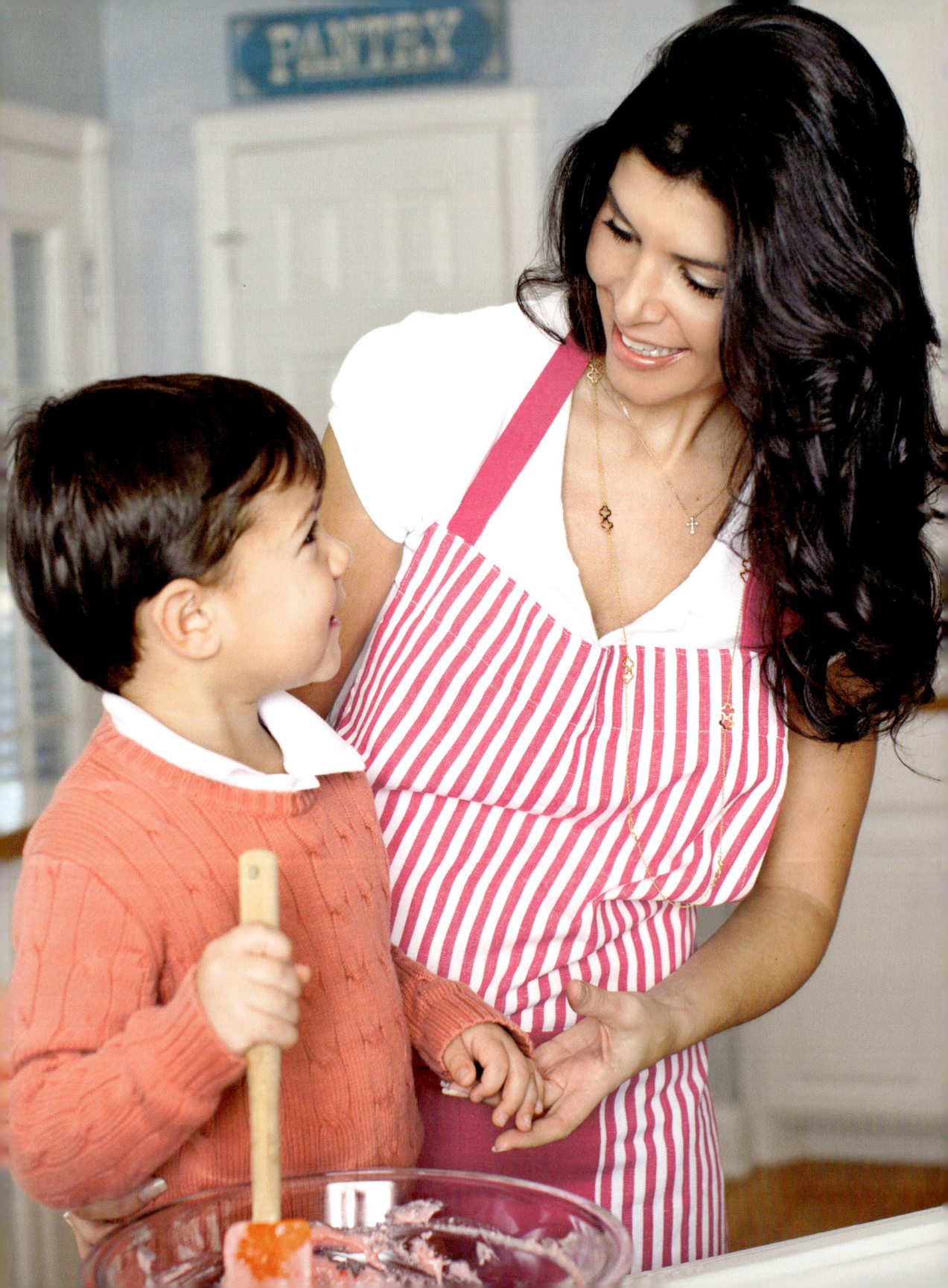

Chapter 11 :

Simply Sinless Snacks

Snack attacks are inevitable, but snack time is a danger zone. In fact, all your hard work can quickly go up in smoke if you aren't prepared to offer healthy, low-fat snacks that take the edge off your appetite.

What follows are some of my all-time favorites, and many are Simply Sinless, which means they're super easy to make.

Simply Sinless "Fried" Zucchini

INGREDIENTS

4 tablespoons seasoned
   breadcrumbs
3 tablespoons reduced-fat
   Parmesan cheese
1 teaspoon cayenne (this is optional,
   but it adds a spicy kick)

2-3 egg whites
2 teaspoons low-fat 1% milk
2 zucchini, cut lengthwise
   and quartered
½ cup marinara sauce
   Nonfat cooking spray

DIRECTIONS

1. Preheat oven to 400 degrees and spray baking sheet with cooking spray.

2. In a pie plate or shallow dish, mix breadcrumbs, Parmesan, and cayenne. In another shallow dish, combine egg whites and milk and whisk with a fork until well blended.

3. First roll the zucchini sticks in the breadcrumb mixture, then the egg mixture, then back to the crumb mixture to coat. Place each stick on the prepared baking sheet and spray with fat-free cooking spray.

4. Bake 15-18 minutes or until golden brown. Serve warm with a side of marinara sauce.

Serves 2.

Simply Sinless Check Me Out Chickpea Cakes *(vegetarian friendly)*

INGREDIENTS

1 can chickpeas, rinsed and drained
1 cup shredded carrots
½ cup seasoned dry breadcrumbs
1/3 cup low-fat creamy Italian
    salad dressing
3 small egg whites

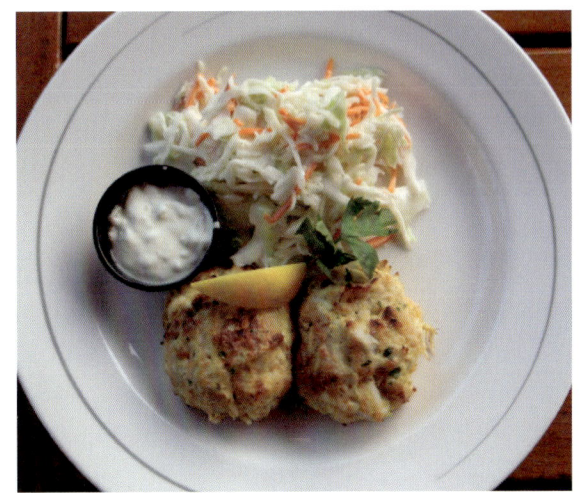

DIRECTIONS

1. Preheat oven to 350 degrees and spray baking sheet with fat-free cooking spray

2. Using a potato masher, mash chickpeas in a large bowl and stir in carrots, breadcrumbs, salad dressing, and egg whites. Mix until well blended.

3. Shape the chickpea mixture into desired patty size and bake 15-18 minutes or until lightly browned on both sides, turning over when halfway through baking time. Serve warm with creamy Italian dressing for dipping.

Makes 4-8 cakes, depending on desired size.

Ham & Cheese Baguette

INGREDIENTS

2   medium red bell peppers
1   loaf whole grain French bread
½   cup fat-free Italian dressing
1   small red onion, sliced thin

6-8 slices lean deli ham (lunch meat)
8   large fresh basil leaves
3 slices reduced-fat Swiss cheese, sliced thin and halved

DIRECTIONS

1. Preheat oven to 350 degrees and spray 13 x 9-inch baking pan with fat-free cooking spray.

2. In a large bowl, beat the cake mix, peanut butter, and Splenda on low until mixture is crumbly. Separate 1/3 cup of the mixture and set aside in another bowl for topping. In the main bowl, add water, egg whites, applesauce, and oil and beat on medium speed until well blended.

3. Spread batter evenly in the prepared pan. In the topping bowl, add chocolate chips, peanut butter chips, and peanuts and mix well. Sprinkle the mixture over the batter in the pan.

4. Bake 38-40 minutes or until inserted toothpick comes out clean. Cool on a wire rack, serve, and enjoy!

Serves 6.

Simply Sinless Mini Pizza Pitas

INGREDIENTS

2 whole wheat pitas, cut horizontally to make thinner for baking

½ cup marinara sauce

1 teaspoon dried basil

¼ teaspoon dried red pepper flakes (this adds a kick, so dial it down to 1/8 teaspoon if needed)

1 cup sliced mushrooms

12 slices cooked pepperoni (usually packaged, not raw)

½ cup thinly sliced green bell pepper

½ cup thinly sliced red onion

½ cup reduced-fat shredded mozzarella cheese

2 teaspoons reduced-fat grated Parmesan cheese

DIRECTIONS

1. Preheat oven to 475 degrees.

2. Place pita halves, cut side up, on prepared baking sheet. Spread marinara evenly over all four pitas and sprinkle with basil and red pepper flakes. Add mushrooms, 3 slices of pepperoni per pita, bell pepper, and onion, then sprinkle with mozzarella.

3. Bake for 5-7 minutes until cheese is melted. Sprinkle each pita with Parmesan and serve hot.

Makes 4 pizzas.

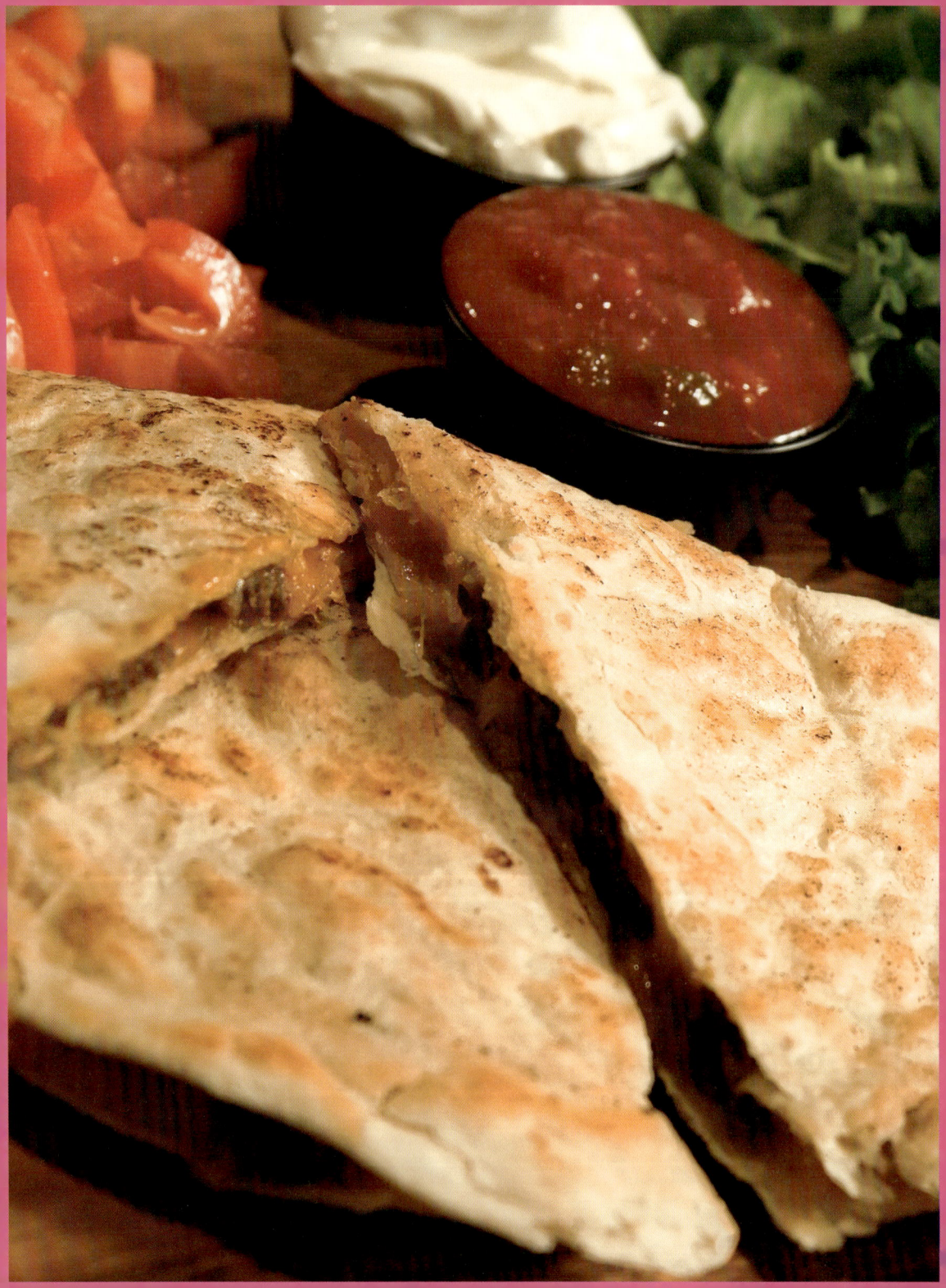

Superfast Southwestern Wedges

INGREDIENTS

2   small whole wheat or vegetable tortillas

1/3   cup reduced-fat Mexican-blend cheese, shredded

½   cup cooked chicken or turkey (lunch meat or rotisserie)

1   green onion, sliced thin

     Salsa to taste (roughly 3 tablespoons)

DIRECTIONS

1. Heat large nonstick skillet over medium.

2. Spray 1 side of tortilla lightly with cooking spray and place in pan, sprayed side down. Top unsprayed side with cheese, chicken, green onion, and salsa. Top with second tortilla and spray top with cooking spray.

3. Cook 2-3 minutes per side, flipping until golden brown and cheese has melted. Cut into wedges and serve hot.

Serves 2-4.

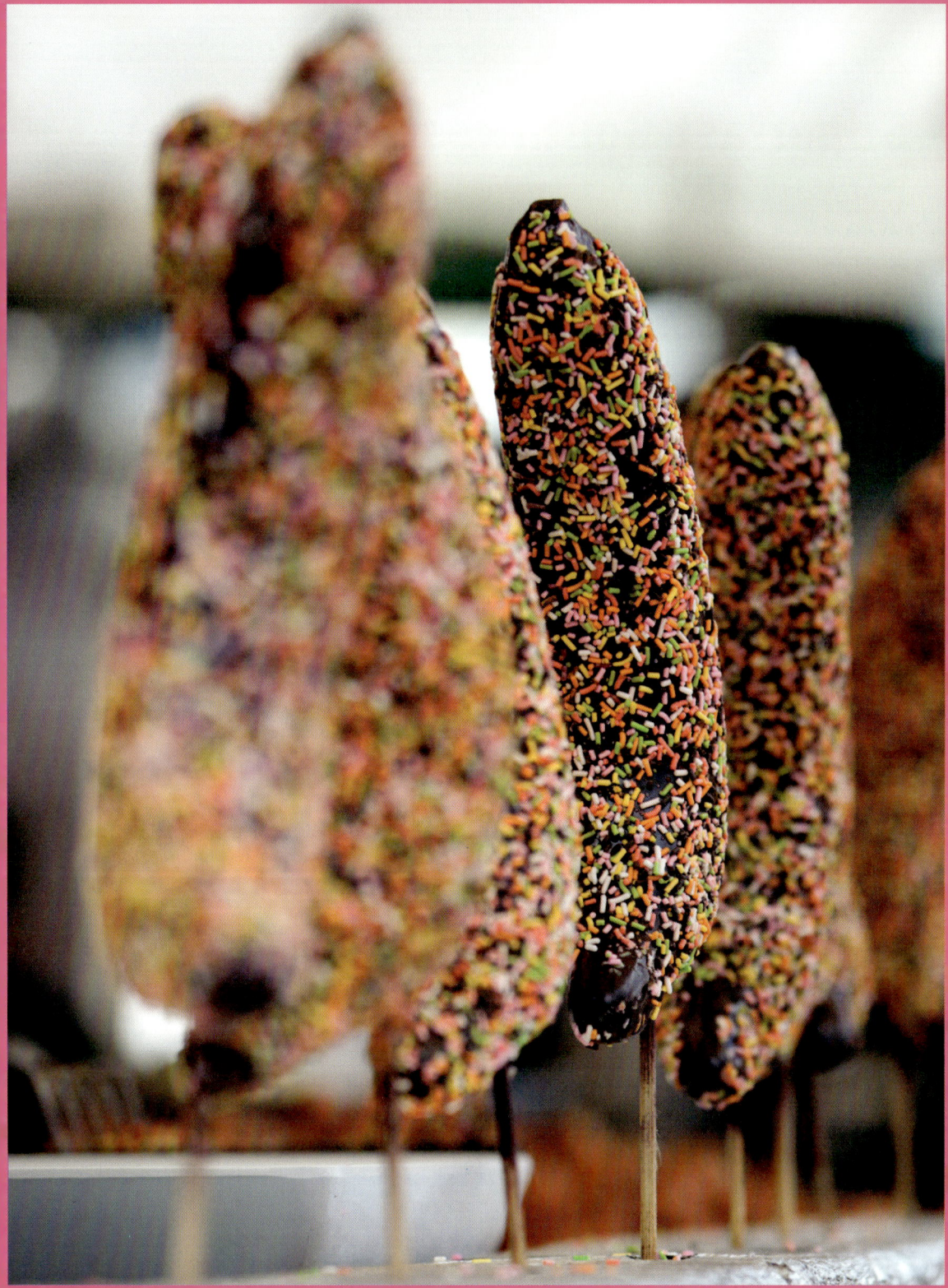

Fast & Fabulous Chocolate Bananas

INGREDIENTS

2   large bananas

4   wooden sticks (typically found
       at craft stores)

2/3 cup granola

Sprinkles and other toppings, optional

½   cup reduced-sugar hot fudge topping
       at room temperature

DIRECTIONS

1. Line a baking sheet with waxed paper and set aside.

2. Cut bananas in half crosswise and insert a wooden stick into the center of the cut end of each banana half. Place on the baking sheet and freeze until firm, about 2 hours.

3. Pour granola into a shallow plate and ensure all large chunks are broken up. Pour the hot fudge topping in a shallow dish or pie plate.

4. Dip frozen banana in hot fudge topping, coating evenly, then transfer to granola plate and turn to coat. Place banana back on baking sheet and repeat with the other three bananas.

5. Freeze chocolate and granola-covered bananas for another 2 hours, until fudge topping is firm. Allow to thaw about 5-8 minutes before serving.

Serves 4.

CONCLUSION

"You can't heal your heart through your mouth." – Tania N. Boughton

It has been a pleasure to share with you both my journey and my inspiration for eating healthfully. Simply put, self-love through self-care allowed me to end the damaging and hopeless cycle of emotional eating that had dogged my every step since I became an adult. The words, "You are fat, you are fat, you are fat" no longer apply to me and they never will again, because I no longer hide behind weight gain, nor do I despair because of it.

I believe self-love can end emotional eating for you, too, and I implore you to break this cycle and do something good for yourself. Part and parcel with this, you will be doing something good for the people you love the most. I like to think of this as self-care at the cellular level.

Finally, remember that I'm in the trenches with you. Every day, I have to recommit to eating well and providing healthy, delicious food for my family. I slip up once in a while – we all do – and I do not hold myself to an impossible standard. But I can and do hold myself to a realistic standard, and at five years and counting, I'm walking, talking proof that *Eating Light, Done Right* works.

I wish you good luck, good love and good food. Oh, and be on the lookout for book two in my Simply Sinless series due to be released in 2013, *Eating Light, Done Right 2…Fast and Fabulous! The Second Collection of Simply Sinless Recipes for the Overworked, Overstressed and Overtired Mom.*

Hugs,

~ Tania

Appendix

with Gym Workouts

Full Body Circuit – MONDAY

Do these exercises below as a series, as many rounds as possible for your allotted time.

EXERCISE	WEIGHT	REPS/TIME	SETS
Squats		45 sec.	
Good mornings		45 sec.	
Lunges		45 sec.	
Step-ups		45 sec.	
Push-ups		45 sec.	
Arm circles		45 sec.	
Dips		45 sec.	
Quadrupeds		45 sec.	
Sit-ups		45 sec.	
Supermans		45 sec.	

Cardio / Core – TUESDAY

If you are capable, run as much as possible, taking walking breaks when needed, but keep moving forward. If you have treadmill access and prefer that modality, by all means use it. If you prefer the great outdoors, map your route ahead of time and try to cover just a little more ground each session.

EXERCISE	WEIGHT	REPS/TIME	SETS
Walk / Run		30-40 min.	
CORE SERIES			
Plank *(prone core hold)*		30-60 sec.	3

Full Body Strength – WEDNESDAY

Multi joint movement

Exercises may be performed without weights for beginners, with light hand weights for intermediate exercisers, and with heavier weights/exercise bands for advanced exercisers.

EXERCISE	WEIGHT	REPS/TIME	SETS
Squat & Press		15	15
Deadlift & Row		15	15
Step-Up & Curl		30	15
Lunge & Lateral Raise		30	15

Cardio / Core – FRIDAY

Intervals

Run for a minute, walk for a minute, repeat for time. If running is not an option, do a comfortable walk for a minute, followed by a speed walk for the next minute. Again, repeat for time.

EXERCISE	WEIGHT	REPS/TIME	SETS
Run/walk intervals		30 min.	
DO THE FOLLOWING CORE EXERCISES IN ORDER AS A SERIES:			
Toe Touches		15	4
Cobras		15	4
Bicycle Crunches		30	4

ABOUT THE AUTHOR

Tania is a full time single mom to two little boys, one of whom has Asperger's syndrome. She also juggles a men's fashion career with J. Hilburn, a long-term relationship, volunteering for her sons' PTA, raising money for the Cystic Fibrosis Foundation and other charities, attending her sons' sporting activities five nights a week, exercising, writing this book, and tending to the daily cooking, laundry, dry-cleaning, dishes and STRESS that come with modern life. You name it, she does it, because she really IS the mom next door!

Tania, who lives in Dallas, Texas, saw what appeared to be a hole in the self-help/cookbook market as she quickly dropped her baby weight and experienced droves of people at the gym asking "How?" As she dug deeper, she realized that while she had made the decision to stop eating emotionally, many of these people had not. Herein lies the groundwork for *Eating Light, Done Right: Simply Sinless Recipes from the Single Mom Next Door.* Drawing on her experience in the military counseling troops on weight control, Tania quickly realized that she loved helping people face the demons within. This turning point redirected her life in a positive direction.

Countless hours in the kitchen later, burning herself on a near daily basis and stubbornly refusing to purchase thousands of dollars' worth of fancy cookware, Tania has transformed numerous favorite recipes from full fat, high-calorie "fat bombs" into easy, light recipes that you don't have to be an "expert at anything" to make. Her approach is frank and light-hearted with the underlying message that if she can do this, anyone can. As she states at the end of nearly every recipe, "Serve hot and enjoy!" Emphasis on **enjoy**!

Index